No More
Secrets

Patricia Gallagher

Copyright page

Library of Congress Cataloging-in-Publication Data
Gallagher, Patricia C1951-
Home Child Care – How To Set Up A Fun And Successful Program In Your Own Home
Revised edition of: Start Your Own At-Home Child Care Business. 1989, Doubleday

Patricia Gallagher,
1. Day care centers – United States. 2. Child care business. 1. Title
    362.7
    This book is a revised edition of *Start Your Own At-Home Child Care Business,* originally published by Doubleday in 1989 and Mosby Lifeline in 1995.

ISBN:1537762079

For information, please contact:
Patricia C. Gallagher
Box 561
Worcester, PA 19490
Telephone: (267) 939-0365
www.patriciausa.com
Cover graphics designed by www.freepik.com

Dedication

To my loving family for their never-ending support

John, Robin, Katelyn, Kristen and Ryan

John's Story

My wife woke up and saw me standing above her, next to the bed. I was dressed, but not in work clothes.

"Trish, there's something wrong with me. . . . I tried to kill my-self. I was driving around. I was going to drown."

Trish got me to lie down; she covered me with a blanket. Then, she called my office and left a message for my boss, telling her that I would not be in for the rest of the week—that things were seriously wrong. She got Katelyn, age14, Kristen, age 12, and Ryan, age 9, off to school, then called my doctor. Robin, age 16, was al-ready on the school bus.

"This is Patricia Gallagher," she said. "I'm John Gallagher's wife. He's been in to see you a few times. Doctor, he needs to go somewhere to have a rest." She continued: "He's been driving around for an hour this morning. I didn't even know he was out of the house. Doctor, something is wrong. Where can I take him?"

On the doctor's recommendation, Trish made arrangements to take me to a hospital where there was a psychiatric unit. It was a beautiful day but, as usual, my mood was totally flat.

"John, do you want to go to Denny's and have breakfast?" "I don't care," I replied.

"Do you want to take a ride?" "I don't care."

The I don't cares were my only response.

As we drove on, I said plainly—almost matter-of-factly—"I'm going to die."

"No, John, you're just stressed," Trish insisted. "You need a vacation." She strained to speak calmly.

As we pulled into the Emergency parking lot, I blurted out: "Take me to the ER. I'm going to die. I took carbon monoxide."

I confessed that, when I went out driving around, at approximately 6 a.m., I had pulled the car over and breathed the exhaust from the back of my car.

She asked how long. I said, "I guess about nine or ten minutes." I didn't want to say anything more than that. I knew she would just try to placate me and tell me everything was going to be okay. For me, I didn't think that things would ever be okay again. So we went into the hospital, hoping upon hope that we would somehow find relief.

As a man in this world of ours, I am expected to hold a job, make enough money to pay my bills, provide for my four children, and be there for my wife. But sometimes, in the hustle and bustle of daily life, all the tasks and responsibilities cascade into over-whelming stress. That's what happened to me nine years ago.

On the outside, everything looked great. I had an MBA, a job as a financial analyst, and a wife and four children. But, on the inside, everything had begun to fall apart. My company was cutting back, and I feared being laid off and rendered incapable of providing for my family. I also feared telling my father and my father-in-law about the possibility of losing my job.

I had a perfectly good job in the Advertising Administration department of a major pharmaceutical company. But, even be-fore the announcement of future lay-offs, I didn't think that was good enough. Recently, I'd started thinking that I should be-come a pharmaceutical sales representative. The people in that department seemed to be the "beautiful people" in the company and, I figured that, if I made it into that elite group, I'd have success.

Come to think of it, I had always felt that I wasn't good enough. I would get good jobs with Fortune 500 companies, but, once on the job, I'd start to think that I wasn't up to par. I would try to follow the adage, "Fake it 'til you make it," but doing so was very stressful for me. I also tried to go with the saying, "Don't let them see you sweat," but, since I was always worried about being fired, I wasn't very good at that either.

Following popular wisdom didn't do me much good.

Life began to overwhelm me. What I didn't know then is that my high degree of worry and anxiety, coupled with the sense of not being good enough, were classic signs of depression.

About two years after my accident, my family and I went to visit my aunt at the New Jersey shore. I asked her about my mother, who had died when I was only nine years old. I really didn't have many memories. I did wonder why God did that to me, have a little boy lose his mother so young. I knew that she was very beautiful. I had seen so many pictures, wonderful pictures, but I really didn't know much about her. I knew that there were many gifts my mother had given me, in my genetic makeup, and I treasure all of them. I know that she had strength in the face of setbacks and that she was very creative. All of the photos showed me that she was very particular about the way her children were dressed and cared for. When she did a job, and when I do, I do it right. I guess we were both perfectionists. My grandparents were Polish and very loving to me. I remember that after my mother died, my grand-mother always stroked my cheek very tenderly. We always had a houseful of relatives there and laughed with our grandfather until our sides hurt. I remember people being very nice to me after my mother died and giving me candy.

During the conversation, my aunt said, in passing,

"Oh, your mother was so good at flower arranging! See that wall hanging over there, Johnny? She made that for me, and I've saved it for forty-five years."

My mother, my beautiful mother had so many talents and gifts. How I wish somebody had told me more about her over the years. I never knew how my mother died. I don't remember her complaining and I don't remember her being sick. No doubt about it now, she must have been terrified about leaving her family. I guess a lot of other relatives knew and never talked about it. I can almost imagine my mother saying, "Johnny, I am proud of you and I love you so much!" How I long to hear those words. I feel connected to my mother in a special way now.

A few hours later, as Trish and I were walking along the board-walk, I started to cry. I cried another time, uncontrollable sobs. I was looking at our wedding picture and so many relatives had passed away. A sadness hit me that would not go away. *That could have been me, another Gallagher missing from the family,* I thought. The thought of how I had almost left my family terrified me now.

"I wish my mother was here," I said. "She's the only one that would know that it's not my fault, that I'm not a wimp."

That's what it had seemed to me—that being depressed was like being a wimp because it meant I was too weak to take charge.

As we walked, moments of depression came flashing back. The first was when I was about 18. I woke up and felt like a massive freight train was running through my head. I never told anybody about it.

The next time I had this frightening experience was when I was 24 years old and out at a club with my friends, dancing and partying. Suddenly, I started feeling strange—not intoxicated, not drunk, but strange. I was sure that somebody had put something in my drink. I went home, feeling dizzy; my head was spinning. When I went to bed, I couldn't sleep. My heart was racing. I felt as if a massive freight train was running through my head again, at a hundred miles per hour.

That lasted for a couple of days. Again, I didn't tell anyone. For many years, I believed that it was all a matter of some prankster putting a drug in an unsuspecting guy's drink. Over the years, though, the same feeling would come back sporadically, when there were no drinks and no possibility of pranksters. And there was no possibility of me being at a club called Uncle Sam's American Flag.

When it came back in 1990, the circumstances were entirely different. I was happily married, with three children and one on the way. But just before my son Ryan was born, I started getting anxious. The symptoms were more intense than the first time, and the time frame was slightly longer—four days.

The first night that this was going on, I asked Trish to call the doctor. It was the middle of the night. He told her that it sounded like anxiety, and said that it wasn't necessary for me to go to the hospital. I kept insisting to Trisha that she had to take me to the ER. The doctor did not give me the required referral to go to the ER. He said, "Just tell him to relax."

The next morning, Trish asked me not to go to work, to just stay home and rest but I insisted on going. I hated to miss work but it was tough going there that day. Once I got there, I found myself completely unable to handle things, and ended up leaving work before noon.

While I was at work for that short time, Trish had invited some of the neighbors over for tea and a playgroup. She told her friends what had happened during the night. Diana, an ER nurse, told her that it was anxiety. The word "depression" had not yet come up.

I was able to take some time off from work and stay home; this seemed to do the trick. But I just wasn't myself. I know now that doctors would describe me as having "no affect." Trisha tried to lift my spirits by involving me in her projects, and then taking a ride to Core Creek Park. I felt like I was just going through the motions. I wasn't able to even have a conversation with her.

After four days off, I returned to work and started functioning normally. Whatever the case, my symptoms went away as quickly as they had come. They did not return until 1998.

In March of 1998, I was working at the same pharmaceutical company as in 1990, but in a different capacity. Now I was a financial analyst. I had been doing a lot of overtime at work, and was starting to feel that my job was over my head. I was stressed out from a long commute and the strain of trying to learn new computer programs.

It was about a year before I jumped. Little by little, month by month, day by day, I was starting to feel different. I was scared, sweaty, anxious, irritated, angry, and so confused.

My symptoms had returned with a vengeance. My condition was worse than ever, and I couldn't seem to shake it.

Many evenings, when I was helping the kids with their home-work, the headache, the racing heart, and the feeling of helplessness would come back. I couldn't focus on helping them.

I remember coaching my daughter's basketball team, and feeling and looking like the living dead. My wife now recalls watching me as I coached, and seeing how timid and uncertain I looked. To both of us, I seemed like the shadow of my former self. Yet, it wasn't constant. I remember being elated when Kristen's basket-ball team won the championship and by all accounts, the home videos look like I was one happy dad cheering from the sidelines.

One night, I was at the mall with the kids, when Kristen asked, "Dad, are you all right?" I felt as if I was having a heart attack, and had to leave the mall. I was afraid I would embarrass my family. I hated the thought of embarrassing them.

Something else started happening. My worrying started to invade my sleep. Sleep became frightening and stressful, then, ultimately, impossible. My initial episode of frenzied sleep paved the way for three solid months of insomnia—something which further incapacitated me.

During that first night of troubled sleep, I experienced a sense of obscuring darkness, followed by a different, more palpable darkness that stirred inside me. I awoke and felt my brain racing in a way that I had never experienced before. It was worse than the time when I was in my twenties, and worse than the time before Ryan was born. I thought to myself, *What is going on? Did I eat something? What is this*? I prayed to God for this foreign and scary feeling to leave me, but it did not. I got up, walked downstairs and turned on the television. My head throbbed and my heart raced. Could this be a stroke? I wondered. Or a heart attack? I began pacing up and down the house, focusing on the agonizing pain in my head and wondering what it could be.

The noise of my footsteps awoke Trish. "What are you doing?" she asked, sleepily.

"I don't know," I responded. My head writhed with pain as I spoke. "I think I have a brain tumor. My head is killing me. It's excruciating."

After a restless night, I still had the throbbing headache from the night before. Though I didn't feel like I could do anything, I went to work.

At work, I felt unable to function. I couldn't concentrate. Everything faded into nothingness and seemed unreal and insignificant, compared to the ever-present, searing pain that was splitting my head in two. My coworkers noticed that I was not my-self. They had no idea just how disoriented I felt.

This time, the symptoms alarmed me. I knew enough to know, by now, that it was something serious that was not likely to just go away. I had been seeing a family doctor for months. I prayed earnestly, "God, please help me with this headache. Please help me go to sleep. Please help me to get to the right doctor. Please help me beat this thing."

My family doctor prescribed several medications as he tried to help me find relief. He also listened patiently, as doctors do, and prescribed yet another drug for anxiety. The drug did not seem to help. I took it for a few weeks and I didn't like the side effects. I went back to the doctor. He reminded me that it takes time for medicine to work. "Give it time," he said.

In my depressed state of mind, I probably was not hearing what the doctor, or anyone else, had to say. My brain was often racing, and I was distracted and impatient. I stopped taking the medicine, not realizing that this could make things even worse. But honestly, the word depression had no meaning to me at the time. I just felt physically sick with headaches being my chief complaint.

What I know now, but did not know then, was that a family doctor may not be equipped to deal with the sort of chemical imbalance that was going on inside of me. At this point, my anxiety had progressed to a serious level. I needed to see a psychiatrist, but did not realize it at the time.

As time dragged on, the unbearable feeling in my head persisted. On one occasion, I went with my wife to a healing Mass, where I pleaded, "Please, God, let this Mass work. Let it take my headache away." But I returned home, still unable to sleep and without relief from the headache.

As time went on, my situation only worsened. In addition to the pain, anxiety surged, and, increasingly, heart palpitations took my breath away. Sleepless nights became the norm, and eating became an undesirable chore. I simply had no appetite. I had lost close to 60 pounds and had gotten into the habit of wearing two sets of clothing to try to hide how thin I had become. Feelings were absent. I could not concentrate, and felt powerless. My wife and kids were supportive and loving, but I was growing frustrated, and so were they.

I tried everything I could think of to deal with the darkness that had descended upon my life. I even went to a neurologist to check for a brain tumor. There was none. Then I went to a cardiologist, who told me it was high blood pressure. From a multitude of doctors, to healing Masses and prayers, nothing seemed to help. I felt betrayed by God, and completely abandoned in my suffering.

I was beginning to have crazy thoughts inside my head, but I didn't share them with anyone. I thought of running in front of a car near my workplace in Princeton, and of trying to drown myself in our bathtub when my wife and kids went on an outing. I even held a knife to my chest at one point, but the blade was dull. I thought of jumping from the roof of the building where I worked.

These thoughts terrified me. I had always been very sensible and logical. After all, my background was in accounting, where everything had to line up evenly. Thoughts like this were torturing me, and nobody knew but me. *Where were they coming from?*

They were absolutely crazy, illogical thoughts. What was happening to me? My thoughts were fractured, frazzled, and clearly not mine. But I still had to do my work and take care of my family, even though I was falling apart, with irrational thoughts echoing through my head. It seemed like life was going on for everybody else. They were laughing, smiling and all was well, but for me, I thought that I was dying and I didn't know what to do about it.

I was the kind of dad that worried about my kids getting hurt, probably known as a "worrywart." I worried about the kids falling from their bikes, running in a parking lot, going out too far in the ocean or falling off the second floor of a railing at a hotel balcony.

Suffering was one thing, but the feeling of isolation and loneliness was another. I felt that no one understood and that no one could help me. I felt hopeless and helpless.

Finally, something inside of me snapped as I drove to work one day. I started to think about going to the bridge. I planned to jump but I couldn't do it. The thought of inhaling gas fumes gave me a sense of peace. I pulled my car to the side of the road, got out of the car, and put my mouth to the exhaust pipe of my car. After a few minutes, I lifted my mouth from the pipe and got back in my car. Somehow in the midst of this decision, I was aware that my link with God, though thin and worn, was still intact. He still had a hold on me. I knew—at least theoretically—that my life was to live, not to take. I didn't want to die. I just wanted this pain to end. I drove home and told my wife what I had done.

I let my wife drive me to the hospital, to continue our desperate search for help. They kept me for one night and discharged me in the morning. A day later, I was admitted again. When I arrived at the hospital that day, my blood pressure was still very high. After several hours being treated in the ER, they decided to admit me for the blood pressure issue and they took me to the cardiology wing.

Soon after I was settled into my hospital room, Trish came in. She stood patiently by the chair where I was sitting, and started showing me a photo album filled with pictures of my kids—kids that I love with all my heart. Interspersed with the pictures were hand scrawled red heart-shaped Valentine cards with paper lace, stickers highlighting birthdays, words in the margins, tickets from concerts, grade school report cards, reminders of involvements with our church's service projects, and little reminders of all of the love I had in my life. A life of former happy memories. Katelyn and Kristen singing the Ave Maria on the altar at church. A baby cradled in my arms. Pictures on the beach. Class trips. Christmas lights. Birthday parties. Photos with the Easter Bunny at the mall. My son with his baseball cap and wiffle ball playing in the Youth Baseball program. Small cherubic faces giving me homemade gifts. How would I ever recapture those moments that had brightened my life? All of the wonderful memories of my "old life" were there. I never thought I would hear "Batter up!" again. I wrestled with so much doubt and believed they were gone forever.

Trish told me that she and the kids loved me and that everything was going to be okay. I had lost faith in myself. I thought,

What is wrong with me? I had tried talking to God and listening to God.

Now, all help seemed remote and I felt so afraid. The life I had seemed to have dissolved, no interest in hobbies, reading mystery novels, driving to look at beautiful houses, or going to flea markets with the family. My mind could not penetrate the heavy fog that blocked all rational thinking. I felt trapped, raw, broken and mentally exhausted in this hospital room. I needed a break.

The pictures were meant to cultivate some feelings of happiness in me. The summer before, my girls had gone to repair a house for a mission trip. A photo of them beaming, with hammers and paint cans in hand, looked up at me. Instead, the photos began hammering away at me and made me feel all the more desperate, convinced that the best was all behind me now. The sadness I felt eclipsed everything in that album.

Then, Trish left the room to phone her mother. She wanted to tell her that I was doing fine and ask her to bring me a pair of shoes. Robin and Katelyn were out with their friends and the two younger ones were at Trish's mother's house.

Alone in my hospital room, I reflected on my loving family, thinking that the best of life was now in the past and could only haunt me. My twisted thinking led me to imagine that they would commit me to an insane asylum, a place I had heard about in movies. The thought terrified me. I wasn't thinking clearly and even said to Trish, "They're not going to kill me, are they?" *Where were these absolutely torturous thoughts coming from? This wasn't me.* I had a world-class wonderful family and a great life, but it all seemed to be crumbling beneath me. At that point, nothing was able to shine through the darkness in my mind. I was stunned about all of this, more like numb, gripped with a doubt that offered no hope.

I looked at the window, which seemed to be calling me, challenging me. I saw the same thing I had seen in the exhaust pipe of my car—a way to end my suffering. I arose from the chair, and approached the window. The raw throbbing in my head had dulled my thought process; I acted without much thought beyond the drive to escape. Numb from everything but pain, I looked down. *I can do it,* I thought. *I will do it.*

I jumped, relieved that the pain would finally go away.

It did not. The descent was frightful; the impact was heavy, obliterating.

When I jumped, I had no idea how high up I was. I didn't know whether I was 1000 feet above the ground or 50. I have been told since then that I fell 40-45 feet, and landed in a cement window well, or—as the ambulance attendant called it—a "viaduct." I think I may have hit the side of the building on the way down.

I heard that there was one eyewitness in the parking lot. I wish that I could talk to that person and find out what really happened. But it took me nine years to want to know—and nine years to go back and stand in front of the window from which I had frantically pitched my body.

I returned to that spot with my wife and my daughter Katelyn in July, 2008. When we got there, Katelyn and I stood in front of the building and stared up at the window together. After my first startled glimpse, I shifted my eyes to the tangible details of the scene—the window well, the cement walkway, the trees—and contemplated the enormity of what had happened.

It struck me then, as now, that I am amazingly lucky to have survived—that it is only by the grace of God that I am not a quadriplegic—or dead. As I stood with Katelyn in front of that window, I pondered the fact that my remarkable family was with me once again in the same place—still with me, despite the intervening an-guish. I prayed to God with gratitude for their presence and my safe-keeping.

I started walking away from the window, then went back— ready to remember and reconstruct the deadly moment.

I flipped in the air and then landed on my legs; they crumbled under me. Rage exploded inside me. I'm still alive, I cried. I could not even kill myself. I lay on the asphalt, bleeding and cursing my survival.

Before I slipped into unconsciousness, I saw Trish's terrified face staring out from the window above me.

Landing on my legs had saved my life, but they were now crushed and broken. The police and ambulance arrived in minutes.

"Cut his jeans off!" one of the paramedics yelled as they slid me onto a stretcher. Voices shouting commands seemed far away, until they faded into nothingness. I fell into unconsciousness.

Shortly afterwards, a doctor awakened me. "Turn your neck," he was saying. "Turn your neck," he repeated, evidently worried that it might be broken. My neck was not broken, I heard him saying, but I had completely crushed both of my legs and sustained head and arm abrasions.

I screamed in agony as he tried to straighten my mangled legs. Several years afterwards, I found out that a nurse had told my wife then that I was not out of the woods—that I still had injuries that were potentially life-threatening. There were bone chips in my blood stream that had caused doctors to worry about infection—an infection that could have done what I had failed to do—end my life.

The next day, my wife and children came to visit in the Intensive Care Unit. They didn't recognize me. When the nurse directed them to my room, they all glanced in and said to the nurse, "That's not our dad." She assured them that it was indeed their father, and that they were in the right room. My head was swollen—like a beach ball, one of the kids later told me. I had a tube in my nose. The kids said that my hair had turned gray. I have heard that sometimes that happens after a shock. I couldn't really talk, but I know that I mouthed the words, "I'm sorry."

Trish's patience through it all has been disarming.

"I want you to know that I love you, the kids love you, we just want you to get better," she said, consolingly. "Whatever you need us to do, we will do for you."

Every day she came in to reassure me, "Don't worry about work, don't worry about money, and don't worry about getting better. As soon as you start getting better, you'll go home and we will all take care of you."

The jump landed me in the mental ward of the hospital, with 24-hour security to keep me from trying to kill myself again. I was there for five weeks, doing rehab for my physical injuries and beginning the process of trying to put my life back together. I needed both physical and mental healing. A psychiatrist was assigned to me. He and I began working on helping my mind, while an orthopedic surgeon began putting my legs back together.

I remember having some strange thoughts while I was in the psychiatric ward. They had aides in the room with me at all times. I was still despondent, and would spend my time thinking of ways to harm myself. I would hold my breath, hoping that would work, or try making myself anxious, in the hopes that I could induce a heart attack.

On one occasion, I had a very strange experience. During this experience, I actually believed that I had died. Perhaps it was a matter of the medication playing tricks on my mind, or perhaps it was my guilt surfacing.

Whatever the case, this is what happened. A nurse was tending to me. As I looked at her, I saw that she had the face of Jesus—the face I had seen in many depictions in books.

Jesus said to me, "Why did you do that? You shouldn't have jumped."

I thought I had died, and that this was Judgment Day. Afterwards, my sister came to visit, bringing magazines and candy. She was being so nice and so compassionate. I felt and thought that I was dead, observing all of this from another vantage point. What a waste! So I played the game. I knew that I had died, but I wanted her to feel that I was still alive.

Then, after my sister left, Trish came in with Ryan. At that point, I was stunned. "You brought my son!" I exclaimed. I had thought I would never see them again. In a state of absolute euphoria, I thought to myself, *Maybe I am alive!*

Trish has since told me that it was at this moment that she left the ward, in despair, to call her mother and say, "Mom, John's never coming back. Something is really wrong with him." But I did. And that moment may have been part of the reason why—for it increased my appreciation of what it is to be alive. It was an epiphany.

I had a few nightmares. I recollected waking up and feeling that I was in a swimming pool and somebody was pouring cement on me. The other was that I was running down a street and somebody was chasing me and I couldn't get away from him.

Everyone visited me faithfully. They sent cards of encouragement and decorated my hospital room with things that they thought would cheer me up—a poster of a horse, stuffed animals and my favorite snacks.

After being discharged, I had to continue doing physical therapy to help repair my battered body. I also had to see a therapist and go to therapy sessions to help repair my psyche. The antidepressants began to kick in, and I started to be able to sleep again at night. My headaches soon faded into memory.

The support of friends and family contributed further to my recovery.

My neighbor rearranged his work schedule so that he could drive me to therapy every day. He lifted my wheelchair into his car, and helped me to get settled into a day program facility. His wife brought meals to my family. They took my son on many outings with them, to baseball games, snowboarding, and amusement parks. They were our lifeline; they knew what had happened, and they gave us tremendous support.

My sister and her family, too, were there for us every step of the way, preparing meals, driving me to appointments, and offering us money to help sustain us. One of her children helped my children with homework while another prepared a delicious chicken casserole.

My wife's family, too, was ever present to help—taking care of the kids, doing odd jobs around the house, and supporting Trisha. My father-in-law was a man of action and he was always coming over, toolbox in hand, grouting the tile, building a bunny hutch or carpeting the patio. My mother-in-law bought new sheets for our bed, left candy on the pillow, and in general was "on the spot" to help wherever needed…anticipating things before she was asked.

All of our neighbors reached out to help, throughout our ordeal, but they did not know what really happened. Several tried to call and visit me in the hospital but I was not where Trisha told them I was. I was in a different hospital, having my mental and physical needs taken care of and could not have visitors other than the family. Someone later told me that it was in the newspaper but nobody let on that they had seen it. Neighbors invited us to picnics and graduation parties that summer but we declined. Trisha just didn't know what to say when neighbors asked questions.

My boss felt really bad about what had happened to me. She wrapped beautiful gifts of books, get-well cards, and a bird feeder and sent them to us. She did many sweet, thoughtful things to tell me she cared. The kids were excited to receive the presents but at that point, I couldn't even manage a thank-you. They expectantly tore away the wrappings, knowing that treasures were inside. The sad truth is that only one person other than my boss contacted me from work. You would think that after more than 11 years, people would reach out. But, I guess because of the nature of the situation, people didn't know what to say or do.

A volunteer visited me in the hospital on a Tuesday morning. She asked me what my favorite dessert was. I told her apple pie. The next day she came back with a little red and white Igloo cooler, with, you guessed it! An apple pie. Not only for me, she brought special desserts for all of the patients. Another volunteer brought a dog. The dog jumped up on my lap. My bones were broken but it was such little acts of kindness that helped me to heal.

I now knew how much everyone loved me and cared. Everyone in our immediate family and our two closest friends did everything they could to help.

I didn't tell my father what had happened, for two reasons. First, he was at the beginning stages of Alzheimer's disease and secondly, I felt a deep sense of shame. It didn't feel manly to have done what I did.

I missed a lot during that time. My daughter Katelyn sang a solo at the junior high, and Robin went to a prom. Kristen had her elementary school graduation, and Ryan was pitching for his base-ball team. Trish told me later how sad she felt to be at the elementary school, being alone at all of the special events, watching the recital, the graduation ceremony and the game—and thinking of me lying in a hospital bed.

There were positive things that came out of all of this, though. When working full-time, I had spent a lot of time at work and very little at home. The kids now had two stay-at-home parents. When I began to feel better, I was able to help Trisha with carpooling and the whirlwind of our kids' activities.

The downside was that my out-of-work status depleted our savings. Disability did not cover our mortgage, insurance and house-hold expenses.

Now, as I was home recuperating, I spent time with the kids, watching movies and plowing through pizza, chocolate cream-filled Tastykakes, ice cream and lots of microwavable popcorn— many nights into the late evening, when they should have been in bed. I really got to know them and their friends, and enjoyed being with them. As I became able to walk and drive, I would take them to school and walk them up to the door. We often came together and gave each other our traditional bear hug which we affectionately called "The Family Squeeze."

I helped Trisha with her "Team of Angels" project, and spent many afternoons with my sister, watching movies and enjoying home-cooked meals. I even took a cooking class at the adult evening school.

However, even though I was on the road to recovery, I was still very irritable and weak from losing nearly sixty pounds and being confined for a time to the wheelchair. I was very worried about where I would work and how I would provide for the family again. Though my family was supportive, it became a lot for me to handle.

After about a year and a half, my wife said we needed to have a serious talk. "I can't do this anymore, John," she said. "We need space. We are going to have to work on all of this apart for awhile." There was a moment of stunned silence and then I responded.

Trish had been going to the monastery of the Poor Clares every day to pray during this overwhelming time. She often sat there in tears, but I did not know this. She had also been going to a family therapist who said,

"Trisha, by the look in your eyes, and from all that you have told me over the past year, I am worried about you. I think you are sinking now, too. Your children need at least one healthy parent. You are going to have to make a very tough decision. I think that you and John need to separate so that you can both work on things and heal separately. You can continue to see each other and plan a date once a week but, for now, it is too much."

Trish asked God to give her the words to say this to our children. She wrote them down in a notebook:

Daddy and I love you all very much but we can't live together right now. We need some 'space' for a while. Daddy will still come over, but we can't all live in the same house right now.

I knew that I had been miserable to live with, and that Trish and I had been struggling to get along with one another. But I did not want to leave them, or to be alone.

I agreed, adding, "It will be better if you go your way. I'll try to heal and get better. You go to therapy and we'll heal separately."

I first went to my sister's house, then I went to live in my father's apartment in Philadelphia. Trish and I maintained our relationship, but it became more of a friendship than a marriage. I was still there often, to remain a father to my kids. We all got together every Sunday and holidays. I never stopped loving my family.

Everything got buried under the rug, all of our emotions, problems and my depression. All of our "sorry-looking baggage" was just packed up and put away. It became a family secret that we hid with all sorts of explanations and excuses. There's that word "embarrassment" again. I didn't want anyone to know. This, in retrospect, was somewhat selfish. I didn't realize the burden this placed on my family.

It probably would have been better if we had just told the truth from the beginning—if we had simply said that I had been suffering with depression after the fear of the downsizing, and that depression had led to a suicide attempt.

If I had acknowledged, earlier, that it was a health problem rather than just an impulsive act of despair, I might have been able to be more forthright. Now I have more of an understanding of what was happening to me. My body's reaction to fearful events had led to a chemical imbalance. The chemical imbalance was related to the stress, and the impaired thinking that resulted from it led to feelings of hopelessness and despair.

I am sure that other people can relate to that. Depression, after all, isn't a new disease in the medical journals!

I believe that we should all be able to talk about depression as we would talk about any other illness. If people were able to do this, the shame of a guilty family secret could be eliminated.

While I was struggling with depression, for the 13 months, before I actually jumped, Trish began writing poems—devotional poems. It was her way of coping, day after day, as she prayed. She called upon a team of angels to help. The first poem was entitled a "Team of Angels for the Overwhelmed." She had never really given a hoot about angels prior to this so my only thought was that it must have been divinely inspired.

She began pairing each poem with a little trio-of-angels pin—something she had started making when the "Team of Angels" concept came to her. She created these pins from materials she purchased at a craft store. Then, after she made pins to go along with her poems, she began making pins by the hundreds, and passing them out to friends, neighbors, and others.

The three angels on the pins were meant to represent peace in our hearts, peace in our homes and peace in the world. And they did, in fact, bring peace to us as a family. The Team of Angels became Trish's lifeline after the tragedy—and something that bridged our family during the ensuing separation—enabling us to heal as a family, and to bond again after we were reunited.

Little by little, almost without even noticing, we did heal. For me, the negativity and irritability began to fade as a more positive me emerged. Medication and therapy sessions slowly gave me back my life. I also took a less stressful job selling clothing. At one point, I worked at a sporting goods store and then sold luxury cars.

I was actually shocked when Trish asked me to come home after a five-year separation. One of our children was going through a tough time, and she needed my help. I, too, wanted this opportunity to be at the center of my family again. The life I had thought was only a memory was beginning to return. Healing is a long process but, little by little, I began to heal, and so did the family.

On February 2, 2006, the day that I returned to live with my family, a new chapter began for us. Trish scheduled a Retrouvaille weekend, something designed to help couples in troubled relationships to heal. At this retreat, we found the tools to bring about healing, knowing that we still had to continue with counseling and to work hard on our marriage.

At around this time, I became actively involved in the Team of Angels project, working with Trish to broaden its reach. During the summer of 2006, Trish and I, together with Ryan and a few of his friends, traveled several thousand miles in a gold van, distributing the pins to those in need. And we began to transform the project into a family business as well as a ministry—one based on the principle of providing encouragement.

The experience of working together on this kind of enterprise brought us closer together spiritually, and gave us the satisfaction of sharing in the creation of something meaningful and sound. Indeed, it seemed that a team of angels had directed our journey from pain to contentment; it had given us a purpose.

On January 20, 2008, yet another chapter began. I read a newspaper story about a high school student who had survived a nine-story jump. What struck me was that he was willing to speak out about his experience. It was then that I began to ask, *Why did I survive? Why did God give me that second chance?*

For some reason, reading that story made me feel not so alone.

You mean somebody else had actually done what I had done. I am a stable guy, level-headed, responsible, and love my family so very much.

What happened to me that night was truly the result of a buildup of stress that so altered my body chemistry, that so literally took me out of my mind, that so made me do something that is literally not comprehensible. I will never forget the feeling of utter despair that I felt at that time. My heart breaks for those who are suffering now. I truly would not wish that on my worst enemy.

How did the idea for writing the book come about? I am not a writer and I never even thought about getting a book published, until the Sunday that I read the four page article in the *Philadelphia Inquirer* about a handsome, popular, 17 year old athlete, who had done what I had done.

I said to Trish, "I am not going to let this happen to **one more** family! This boy is telling my story." I asked her to call our three daughters over for a Sunday dinner. I told them that I was going to write a book and call it *"Don't Jump!"* I asked them if they would each write a chapter. They were shocked. My son lived at home with us, so all four kids were there for dinner.

Trisha passed around the *Philadelphia Inquirer* article and they all read it, or least they started to. They scanned it and laid it down. Perhaps, it was too sad or just too much to absorb. I noticed that none of them read it like my wife did, sobbing throughout. Trish cried as she read each page and said, "John, I never knew you felt all of these feelings." When we each wrote our chapters, it was the first time that we had insight about how this event affected each family member. Many of my notes were on scraps of paper, handwritten on lined notepads. I told my ideas to Trisha and she encouraged me. Then while on my breaks at work, I tried to flesh them out and make sense of all of my ideas. When I told my customers that I was thinking of writing a book, they all said they would want to read it.

Some people warned me that it would be really hard for me to relive all of this and perhaps, I should just forget all about the past and move forward. I certainly never really wanted to be in the limelight, especially for this topic. But if it raises awareness, I am up for the challenge, and committed to doing something about it.

At times, I was nervous about doing this. I was reluctant to share the details. *What would people think of me? How will I ever get another job if I go public with this?* But then I remembered what I had felt like. I told one person and then another. Once I did that, it be-came easier and I found that people were interested in my story.

I wanted to make a difference. My depression taught me that. I remembered my shattered spirit in 1999, the shock of the tragedy on my own family. I knew that this project was more than about me. It was God guiding me, to look at my life through a spiritual lens, and find a lesson of faith and trust through the event. It was as if God was saying to me, "John, you are not weak because of what you went through. You are strong." We started our own non-profit corporation, The Team of Angels Program, which is all about helping families. God saved me and I believe that there are thousands of families that need to know that they are not alone. The work is both satisfying and challenging.

Every time that Trisha and I speak to a group, we learn more about each other. People ask questions and as I answer them, Trish gets a little glimmer of how painful life really was for me at that time. I hear her innermost feelings as she shares with the audience. This is not what I would have planned for my life but hopefully, I can be a voice of hope for someone else.

My four children, now ages 18, 21, 24 and 26 have been guests on radio and television interviews. I am so proud of them. They are all studying psychology in college and I know that they will use their life experiences and compassion to make a difference in the world. I now fully understand that depression brings pain and disruption, not only to the person who has it, but to the whole family. I also know that bringing all of this out in the open may feel uncomfortable for them. So as much or as little as they want to be involved is fine with me. I am so grateful for their love and support. I have a grateful heart that God saved my life and I am able to enjoy life with my family. I want to make the most of the second chance I have been given.

When I decided to speak about my experience, the same *Philadelphia Inquirer* reporter that covered the story about the young man who brought me out of the shadows to tell mine, called for an interview. He asked when I was planning to speak next and by chance, it was that weekend. He came with a photographer and our story was featured on Good Friday, 2008, on the front page of the *Philadelphia Inquirer*. The headline read, *From truth, a way back.....Speaking of suicide restores a man and his family.* It included three photos and a good size news story.

Something very curious happened and I still don't quite understand it. The *Philadelphia Inquirer* is a major newspaper, with a very wide circulation. The article was on the front page......but nobody that we knew contacted us. Nobody called from our old neighborhood. Our relatives didn't call, nor did our friends from past associations, nor from our former church congregation and clubs. We were puzzled. I think the subject of suicide and depression carries such stigma and talking about it makes people uncomfortable. I can understand that completely. I probably would not have reached out to another family. You just don't know what to say, so you say nothing.

But something very amazing happened. Strangers called. People we didn't know looked us up and emailed us or called on the phone. We received many letters, all encouraging us and thanking us for putting a face on the families suffering with depression. They told me I was brave or that I had guts.

They told me about their experiences with depression. They shared that they too felt empty, sad, like nobody cared about them, or worthless.

I work in a clothing store on the Philadelphia Main Line. My employer, Joseph A. Bank, is a pricy retail clothier whose clientele live in affluent neighborhoods, drive expensive cars and seem to be on top of the world without any problems. The day following the *Philadelphia Inquirer* article, several men came into the store to speak to me. They were not all customers but people who wanted to acknowledge that they were personally touched by the newspaper article. They took me aside and thanked me. They thanked me for telling "their" story. They asked me questions and whispered their secret fears, with candor. "John, I don't even feel like watching football any more. I just don't have any energy," one well-dressed man said. "Do you think I should go on medicine?"

Men of diverse backgrounds including a bank president, rabbi, police officer, college student, a few well-respected community leaders, and even two young returning Iraqi war veterans confided their concerns about themselves or their loved ones. They shared about a child with an eating disorder, panic attack or obsessive compulsive issue. One shared about his son serving time in jail for a crime committed when he stopped taking his medication for bi-polar and robbed a mini-mart.

When Sean Andrews, a football player for the Philadelphia Eagles, spoke out to the media about his bout with depression this past season, I was contacted by a public radio station to offer a commentary. Men may be consoled to know that statistics indicate that an estimated 6 million men in the United States have a depressive disorder, but most don't even know it and don't reach out for help. (National Institute of Mental Health)

Unexpectedly, and quite by accident, I became a "support person" for family, friends and even strangers who ask me about medication and talk therapy. I tell them that it takes courage to ask for help, and that it is a strong man, not a weak one, that admits that he wants to get to the root of his feelings of anger, irritability, pessimism and agitation.

Over the years, Trisha brought up the topic of what had happened to me on that beautiful April evening, and I would say, "I don't want to think about that. It's too painful." Sometimes, I would be in such denial that I would say, "I was never depressed. I just had a chemical imbalance." That's true, I did have a chemical imbalance but I also had depression, which is hard for most men to admit. And prior to the depression onset, I had anxiety.

I have now committed my life to helping other "real families with real depression" and specifically "real men with real depression." I feel like a sack of bricks has been lifted from my back, now that I am being open about what happened to me.

My message is that depression is a treatable disease and it can happen to anyone, whether you are a CEO, a Brigadier General, a firefighter, or a priest. I am certainly no expert but after living through this, I want to dedicate my life to educating people about the causes, symptoms and treatments. I want to raise awareness and share my personal story openly. If it happened to me, it can happen to anyone!

I came to the conclusion that God spared me for two reasons: so that I could heal and be a father for my kids, and so that I could help other families deal with comparable experiences. My family and I learned the hard way that hiding this kind of truth is unhealthy and unnecessary. Once I came to this insight, I began thinking that sharing our story might help others break out of this pattern of self-imposed suffering. And that is just what is happening: we are reaching out to others, and giving them the comfort that comes from openness and acceptance.

Recently, a journalist who was working on a national magazine story contacted me. She asked if I thought I had found my vocation. She asked me to explain how this event was life changing. I had to be honest and tell her that the decision to talk about all of this was a tough one to make. I know my book is not a "masterpiece" but it is an honest account about a family man, a "normal kind of guy", John Gallagher, who grew up in Philadelphia, and just planned to be an accountant, certainly not a writer or spokesperson for mental health issues. A person who wondered over the years about the reason his life was spared on that fateful April evening. She even sent a photographer out to our house to take pictures to accompany the proposed article.

Although, that particular article never made it into the national magazine, it confirmed that our story is mainstream enough for publication.

Imagine my surprise when I got a call from *Esquire* magazine for an interview!

I guess the biggest shock was when a Producer from the Dr. Phil Show called Trisha and asked us to share our story. To be considered as guests, they wanted to include the whole family. Two of our children said they were not ready for that. I certainly respect their feelings and appreciate so much, whatever our children are comfortable doing.

I recently spoke at an in-service meeting for the staff at a psychiatric hospital. Also in attendance were a group of patients from their outpatient day program. Many folks came up to me and said how nice it was to hear from someone who had once "walked in their shoes." They told me that it gave them hope that they too could feel better. They felt frustrated because many people thought that they should just "snap out of it" or "pull themselves together."

Now that I have begun speaking out, I find people coming forward to thank me, with a gratitude that is sincere. (I must admit that I have never had so many ladies hug me.) Most are dealing with depression in their own families. Most express the sense of relief that honest dialogue brings.

Reaching out to others has helped our own family to heal. Instead of hiding, Trish and I are reaching out to others by sharing the truth about the pain we went through. Our children, too, have spoken their stories.

I never would have chosen the path of pain I have walked. But now, I can see how that path served to strengthen our family bond and to deepen our appreciation of the spiritual side of life. I am living proof that, no matter how bad things get, there is always a road towards healing, and a plan for our lives. God indeed, works in mysterious ways! Our family's journey is proof of that.

Editor's Notes

I came to know the Gallaghers by an interesting fluke: I had taken a job in the men's clothing store in which John worked. The article about John's attempted suicide, it turns out, had appeared in the Philadelphia Inquirer three months before I arrived on the scene. I became intrigued with John's story, and impressed not only with his courage but his incredibly optimistic outlook. What struck me most clearly about John was his sense of relief in being freed of the burden of secrecy.

I became captivated by the story of the Gallagher family. I saw how they had come together at this important juncture, and how they were finding a way to heal as a family unit. It wasn't long before I met Trisha. We had an immediate affinity, and she soon invited me to take on the role of editor. I was thrilled.

I must say that it has been a pleasure to be involved in this project. I have gotten a full sense of what this amazing family has gone through and what they have learned. Their story illustrates the importance of families being open about depression. It shows how unnecessary it is to hide the truth, and how healthy it is to break the silence. Theirs is a compelling story about a family's courage, awakening, and ultimate triumph; it is truly a love story.

Ellen Bluestone, Editor
ellenbluestone2004@yahoo.com

Patricia's Story

About 13 months before the tragedy, my husband had come home from work with tears in his eyes. He sat next to me on our bed. With his head bent down, he sadly said, "I have three to six months to find another job."

"In the company or outside," I asked.

"It doesn't matter. I just have to get another job," he said resolutely.

At this time our house was on the market. We were planning to move to a house that we had seen that was a little bigger, a little nicer, and a step up from where we lived. It had five bedrooms, a pool and an in-law suite. We were excited because with the way John had figured out the mortgage refinancing, it would only be a slight increase over what we were currently paying. We could handle it and felt it would be a better investment for resale in the future. So even though at times our family resources were somewhat strained, we weren't concerned.

This was the day that he got the news—your days are numbered here. There had been lots of talk about a corporate reorganization and the possible dissolution of his department.

That morning, he had been called into a meeting with a representative of the Human Resources office. John's boss was a kind woman who always sent gifts home to our children for the holidays. Her mother, had even made doll clothes for our girls. She liked John and knew that he had to provide for his family and she had been his supervisor for close to ten years. I am sure it was not an easy conversation for her to have with John, but her department had to cut back. She had no choice but to follow the wishes of her higher-ups, and prepare her employees for possible job losses.

"John," she said, starting out positively, "I know that you are not happy in your position. Where do you think you would fit in the new organization?" However, the conversation plummeted as she added, "This department is probably going to go. We all need to start looking for new jobs. You probably have three to six months to find other employment." John was devastated.

Although, there was no mention of actual firing or a severance package, the message that John heard was that after eleven years of corporate loyalty, he was disposable. He interpreted this as meaning that he was "dead wood", a 48-year-old guy that was as expendable as a light bulb.

The night he gave me the news, he lamented, "I wonder how we'll make it? You don't work, and how am I ever going to get a good job at close to 50 years old? Nobody will hire me when they can hire young kids who will work for much less." Then he added firmly with tears in his eyes, "*I don't want you to tell anyone. It's too embarrassing.*" Through the pools of tears, he said, "*I guess we will make it somehow, but it is so scary.*"

"John, don't worry," I said. "We can move out to a rural area where it isn't so expensive. We don't have to live in this house. We can sell this and get a place for half the cost of our $1900 a month mortgage." Although, that payment seemed very steep, I respected John's business acumen and always trusted his financial decisions. We had recently refinanced for a fifteen year rather than a thirty year mortgage. Payments would be higher now but our pay-off would be less interest paid over the long run.

He was adamant about one thing. "I don't want to move 'down'. I worked so hard all these years so our kids could live in a nice area. I could never tell people the real reason if we have to move." We loved our comfortable lifestyle, our excellent school district, and our neighborhood. We had been here for years—cherishing all the happy memories of Easter egg hunts, family campfires, block parties, mom and tot playgroups and couples getting together for Saturday night dinners—knowing that somebody was always there to help in an emergency was comforting.

I told a couple of close family members about the impending job loss. My parents were there to support me. But, due to a complete denial that it was happening—or to disbelief, or pride—John himself did not confide in anyone. I thought it odd that he did not seem concerned about the impending deadline of August 31st. I asked him what he was going to do. "Nobody has said anything. I am just going to keep going in to my office," he replied.

Throughout the fall, we kept busy with sports activities, going to yard sales, selling Beanie Babies, and doing homework. We transferred our three girls from private school to a public school. They were all okay with that because most of the neighborhood kids went to Council Rock. I clipped coupons and tried to save money in any way I could. My father had always told us to save a "nest egg." Oh, how I wish that we had listened to him.

I scrambled around, trying to find an old teaching resume and any papers related to teacher certification. *Maybe I can substitute teach. That will at least help out. But I would have to get a better-paying job,* I thought. But we both knew that substitute teaching would never even begin to cover our expenses.

We brainstormed about our options. Should we downsize, sell our house, and move to a rental property? Explore home business or franchise opportunities? John was always good about analyzing the pros and cons of any decision. He usually spread a large sheet of paper on the dining room table and analyzed things from many different angles.

He thought that the best idea would be to network within the company. He scoured the listings for intracompany positions in the tristate area. Finally, after a few months, he called me from work. "I have great news. I got a new job, and it pays the same amount." He was offered a new position within the company, on the same level. He was excited about it. No more searching. That night, we sat in a McDonald's restaurant and talked about it.

Seemingly, our worries were over.

But that night he couldn't sleep a wink, and became very anxious. He finally admitted to me his concerns. "I can't work for that

lady. It would be worse than where I am now—like jumping from the frying pan into the fire." He declined the job.

My friend, Marcie, sent us a huge box of books, like *Career Starters, Whose Hiring Who* and *What Color is Your Parachute?* I read through them all, highlighting anything that I thought would help. John diligently read the newspaper for job leads, mailed resumes, and started arranging interviews.

At my urging, we went to two job search sessions at the library. The sight of fifty middle-aged men lamenting their employment woes depressed him even more. It was hard trying to launch a job search while trying to maintain the job he had, especially when his spirits were waning. He continued to work hard at his present job, hoping for a reversal.

He wondered, "If I really work hard and master some of the new contract processes and computer programs, would they reconsider?"

I was concerned. While on a vacation with my parents, we attended a religious retreat at the local church. I hung onto the hope that a spiritual solution was close at hand. The six-month deadline had come and gone. John just kept going into work as usual.

During this initial six-month period, he was beginning to feel excluded. Less important projects were given to him; to him, they seemed like busy work. He told me, "I'm not getting invited to meetings. I'm not part of the team. Nobody wants to bother with me, and I don't have anybody to eat lunch with." Whether that was in fact true, or the darkness of depression coloring his perception, that was his reality.

He called me frequently throughout the day and asked if any employment recruiters had called for him. He also asked me to make exploratory phone calls for him. I wrote thank you notes for him after every interview.

I think the discouragement of the midlife blues came upon him. He looked around the workplace at the DINKS (Double Income No Kids)—his young, mid-twenties competitors, without kids and family responsibilities. There were also lots of very bright interns from local Ivy League schools who were happy to work there for the experience and the opportunity to have a foot in the door for a job after graduation.

John lamented:

"Trish, everybody there is so capable, attractive, and technologically savvy. They can work long hours, and they know all of the new software programs. I'm 48; they run circles around me. Who is going to hire me when all of the young kids know so much about technology and are willing to work overtime?"

Around this time, the company changed its dress code to business casual. This was a significant change, because John's identity and self-esteem were tied to dressing up in a suit. Casual clothing made him feel less himself, less important. This was yet another blow to a man whose confidence in his work skills had already diminished. It got to the point where John needed his spirits lifted daily. "John, it's all going to work out. God has a plan for us," I would say. But I was scared, too.

Our oldest daughter, Robin, was about to have a Sweet Sixteen party. It was December and, I thought back to 1982, the year she was born. I recalled the image of a confident John beaming as he held his first baby. He had bought the obligatory pink-bowed cigars and had taken them to work to pass around. Now, I couldn't ask for any help in planning this special event; he couldn't handle doing homework with the kids, or even sitting and enjoying a movie. He was emotionally spent from worry.

In January, the headaches began. We thought of possible causes, such as hair spray getting into his scalp, food allergies, or a cold that settled in his head. Every evening, he came home from work and went right to bed, but he never fell asleep. He just needed to lie down. I placed warm compresses, cold compresses, and heating pads on his forehead, anything to try to alleviate the pain. But nothing seemed to help.

He wanted desperately to clear up the mystery of the headaches. "John," I told him, "it is stress. You just need a break. Just tell Human Resources that you're sick, and stay home for a few days."

But he answered, "I can't do that. The auditors are coming in and, besides, if I'm out, all of my work will be there when I get back. The other departments need my reports."

He went to our family doctor for the excruciating headaches, and went daily to the nurse at work to check his blood pressure. The doctor warned, "You have high blood pressure and dangerously high cholesterol."

He began to obsess about food, wondering what he could and could not eat. My ideas of eating grains, fruits and vegetables got him upset. "If I eat like that, I'll weigh 90 pounds," he complained.

In February, we attended a family party. He talked about headaches and food for four hours. Family members gave him their ideas on how he could get better. But he could only focus on his eating dilemma. He would discuss it with anyone who would talk about it. Food had become an obsession. *What can I eat for dinner? What am I allowed to eat?* Everything revolved around eating. The rest of the family was becoming stressed.

He began to wear two layers of clothing, so people would stop asking him why he was getting so thin. He bought several pocket-sized calorie counting books at the supermarket checkout counter. He checked out large hardcover medical books from the library, and went daily to the gym. He drank ENSURE, and listened to meditation and relaxation tapes. He was losing weight. He was 6'3" and had weighed 220 pounds. He was down 40 pounds, and worried sick about it.

"I am praying so much, and God won't help me," he complained. I was making daily visits to church myself, praying for something good to happen.

I felt like a widow, managing carpools, homework and sports schedules. My schedule changed, too. I stayed downstairs until 4 a.m., trying to teach myself computer skills, while drinking tea and listening to country music. I cleaned and washed floors, and did laundry in the middle of the night. I couldn't sleep because I was worrying about John and, at the same time, attempting to get a business off the ground. When I finally did come upstairs, he would ask "Was I asleep when you came into the room?" I was so exhausted myself, I did not remember. He lay awake, night after night, sometimes reading to try to fall asleep, but without much success.

I crawled into bed and then within minutes, moved my comforter and pillow to the floor. I started sleeping on the floor with a few quilts because he was so restless. I often had to take two or three Tylenols to fall asleep because my mind was racing, too.

I would no sooner get to sleep when John would be getting ready for work, and I would be waking the kids up for school.

His workday began at 5:30 am. He showered, dressed and drove the girls to the bus stop. Then he would fight traffic for what would often end up being a 90-minute commute. He felt frustrated when the girls would oversleep and miss the bus and he would have to drive them to school.

Working under stressful conditions, bleary-eyed from lack of sleep, frustrated by traffic and the morning routine at home, he was cracking from the pressures.

We were searching for answers for what was happening to John. I just wanted to make him happy again. On his birthday, January 7th, I had an idea. The radio and tape player in John's car had stopped working. He had a long ride to work, and he counted on listening to music to keep his spirits up. I could see that he was sinking lower and lower.

"John, let's go look for a new car. If we leave now, we can get there and have a half hour to spare before the dealership closes." I rushed in to the showroom, with a plan in mind. I went up to a car salesman and said, "We'll take the black Nissan Altima." I added, "We don't need to test drive it—and we need to drive it home tonight." I wrote out a home equity check for $16,000. The salesman was in shock. It was the easiest sale he had ever made.

I knew something was seriously wrong, though, because John did not have any reaction to my impulsivity. He really did not seem excited about the new car. It wasn't like we had money in our budget for such an expenditure. I was just desperate to do something that would cheer him up, something that might bring back the "old John", my husband of 23 years.

Now, I knew that John had a radio that worked and a new car that would make him feel successful. I naively thought that this might be just what he needed to get over this latest hurdle—that this would boost his spirits. I needed the car to boost my spirits, too. I had an interview the next day, with a radio talk show host that I wanted to impress. I "had" to have a new car, didn't I? John's car had missed the state registration deadline. What if I got stopped by the police with the lady in the car? That would have been so embarrassing. The old car was illegal to drive with the expired inspection sticker, and the last thing I needed was for a police officer to give me a citation while driving the talk show host. The interior of my mini-van looked like a landfill and smelled of sweaty sports gear.

He began to blow little things out of proportion. When my daughter had the flu, he worried that she had meningitis. Going to the Sunday flea market, which had always brought him so much joy, would tire him out and make him upset. Going to have his picture taken for his auto license renewal was stressing him out.

At work, the thought of the auditors checking his work became too much to bear. He felt anxious about contracts. He fretted about getting the required signatures; he was worried that he might not have done that before paying the vendors. The prospect of learning new computer programs and taking advanced training sessions was overwhelming.

He couldn't concentrate—at home or at work.

"How can I do all of this—do my job, find another job, pore over classified ads, and do the taxes—and take care of the house and the kids?" he asked, with tears rolling down his face. "I feel like a rubber band is wrapped around my head. Something's wrong with me. Is my forehead bulging out? It feels like there's blood swelled up in my head. How do you know if you have a brain tumor?"

The medical encyclopedia next to his nightstand added fuel to his worst fears. He thought he might be dying.

Yet, the word depression never even came up for us. His health anxieties merged with his work anxieties.

"You have to get me out of there, Trish. They're killing me. People aren't nice. I need to be with nice people. The traffic is unbearable. My head hurts so much."

Several times a day, he called, talking this way and pleading for help.

There were several things that did not seem normal, at this time. We went to a friend's radio show and he was very reserved on the ride there and back, not even able to make any conversation with me. Our oldest daughter was invited to a prom. He couldn't share in the excitement. He didn't even try to be friendly with the boy's parents, when they came to take pictures.

Weekends were no longer fun. We drove around, taking rides, but he was not himself. The musical audio tapes he used to enjoy no longer soothed him. He didn't enjoy doing things with the family. He snapped irritably and inappropriately at the kids. Things were tense and confusing for all of us.

I was mad at him because he was getting very snappy. I told him he needed to contact Dr. Lily, a therapist, for help. He agreed to go. We both called her answering machine and left several messages. She said she no longer worked with our health plan. I made three calls asking other recommended therapists to see John. I seemed to be getting the runaround. I finally found a therapist that had an opening, but his fees were not affordable and he was not in our healthcare network I called another agency, and made an appointment. I wanted John to see a psychiatrist right away. They said you had to have an intake appointment first. That was scheduled, but sadly John never went...John jumped before that date.

John heard the echo of fear in all parts of his life.

What if I can't find a job?

What if we have to move from this house?

What is going on with my headaches?

During a one-month period, he went, repeatedly, to the family doctor and the doctor at work. Biofeedback and a massage were recommended. The company doctor recommended a therapist who was affiliated with the company Employee Assistance Program. John went to her, and focused on the headaches.

On the second visit to the therapist, he came home much earlier than expected. He had only stayed for a few minutes, because he said she didn't know much about headaches.

I then called and made an appointment for both of us to attend a therapy session with her. I told his therapist about the critical job situation which I felt was the cause of the stress and personality changes. She was shocked. She exclaimed, "John never mentioned anything about that to me!"

By now, John was sick of going to doctors. He was sick of feeling down. It wasn't only the wintry January weather. Nothing made him laugh, not videos, our dog or funny stories.

"I've been to my regular doctor twenty times, my work doctor, at least ten times, a neurologist, a gastrointestinal physician, a headache specialist, a stress therapist, a psychotherapist, a massage therapist, and a chiropractor. I've taken all this medicine to sleep and for anxiety. Nothing's helping me. Maybe I should go to the hospital", he sighed.

I didn't see how this would help. "Why do you want to go to the hospital, John?" I asked.

"They might be able to find out why I can't sleep. I feel worse.

I don't like the side effects of the medicine. There's no improvement with this medicine."

"John," I asked, "why are you going to the doctor and the nurse at work so much? It's just stress. You need a rest. You have to rest. We need to take a vacation. My parents will watch the kids." He told me I didn't understand corporate life. "Trish, it's been so long since you worked at AT&T. You don't remember what it's like. You have to keep going in whether you feel good or not," he said.

We had great kids, healthy, cute, smart and kind. Our house was comfortable, and we had a loving extended family. There was always a lot of activity in our home. We had a dog that looked like Lassie, several rabbits, and kids always running in and out the front and back doors. We had lots of fun as a family. Our weekends were filled with our favorite activities, looking at the decorated models of sample houses and going thrift-shopping or as we called it thrift-hopping. We had lots of great friends. For the past decade, John's company offered us a great benefit package, and financial security. He seemed to be a guy who had it all!

He still couldn't sleep, and was losing weight rapidly. Work was hard, home was stressful, and the headaches were excruciating. A couple of times in recent years, we had gone to the hospital because John felt he had something caught in his throat. I remember the first time that happened. We were at a gala event at his company's holiday party. We were "dressed to the nines" and having a wonderful time. Suddenly, John started choking and saying he had to go to the hospital. Upon examination in the ER, there was no "chicken caught in his throat." It was probably related to anxiety, although at the time, we did not know anything about that. That happened several times, once resulting in an overnight stay at the hospital.

We sometimes talked about the idea of him quitting the job, selling the house and "moving down." But our feeling was that, in mid-year, it would add more stress to sell a house, uproot the kids and be without a job. Our daughter was unhappy in her new school, and we arranged for her to go back to her former school. Our third-grader's homework assignments often went unsupervised. I couldn't even get it together to have a neighborhood kids birthday party for him in March. We waited until June to celebrate it.

In March, our daughter had an important issue about a date for another prom. It killed me not to be able to discuss it with my husband. I knew he wouldn't be able to handle it.

As time went on, he didn't enjoy things anymore. He was extremely anxious about routine activities, such as being the assistant basketball coach for Ryan's team—things that under, normal conditions, he loved to do. I thought that a trip to the roller skating rink would cheer him up. He laced up his skates without any enthusiasm and gliding to the music didn't work either. I wanted a comeback...a comeback of my husband, but things felt different these days.

He was always worried about some ailment, and experienced sweating, nervousness, headaches, stomach pains, swelling in the head, insomnia and weight loss. His hands were fidgety, his body jerked in his sleep, and his heart—he said—felt like it was beating out of his chest. That was the main thing—the physical ailments. He was sure he had a brain tumor.

"Please, John," I begged," take some time off from work. It's too much for you right now."

His increasing upset was especially clear in his coaching. I could see that rushing to practices was unnerving him. Watching him from the sidelines, I could see that he looked wiped out, skinny, and unhealthy. He no longer had the strong, athletic presence that I knew my husband to have. He seemed timid. His face looked sweaty.

Everything was either failing or falling onto my lap—paying bills, running sports carpools, driving to CCD classes, and taking care of social activities. Family routine was far from normal. I was so worried about him.

I felt like I had a fifth child. I needed to nurture and encourage him, assuage his worries about health problems, and assure him that I could start a business that would make money. It created so much pressure.

I kept telling the kids every night, "Go to bed. I need to talk to Daddy." We would talk. We would hop in the car and go to a shopping center parking lot and talk. I made up all kinds of errands for him to run with me, to try to keep him active. He was discouraged, and mentally and physically exhausted. Every morning, he would say, "I didn't get any sleep."

I confided in my mother and two friends about my worry over John. My mother recognized what she saw as signs of depression.

One friend, a former nurse in a cardiac unit said, "You have to get him out of that workplace no matter what. You don't want to be visiting him in Temple Hospital after he has a heart attack."

My sister said, "You better get him some help or you're going to be a widow."

In mid-April, he called from work. "They said that everything is safe with my job."

My mother said, "I guess he's really relieved."

"No, mom," I answered. "You don't understand. His emotions were flat. He said it like it was just a fact. It didn't seem to matter to him at all."

On April 27, John called from work and said, "I'm going to go in and talk to Human Resources about quitting." When he arrived home, he was very distressed and said, "I didn't talk to them."

"John," I said, "I'm going to call them now. What's the phone number?"

"Trish, what are you going to say?" I answered:

"I'm going to present them with a request for some kind of package that would be win-win. Let's think of a solution that would meet their need to replace you and also give you a salary for six to nine months—with benefits for the kids' braces and medical. I'll tell them we need security while we work on starting a home business. I'll ask someone to meet us at Denny's restaurant on Route 1 to share ideas."

I started to dial, but John resisted. "No, Trish, I'll talk to them. That would be gutless if you called for me. I'll talk to them in the morning."

Under these strained conditions, the job of keeping up with the activities of four kids, worrying about the impending job loss and John's waning spirits, it started to become a strain for both of us. One night, the routine started to break down. John was at Ryan's Little League baseball practice. Robin and Katelyn were there, too. Kristen was at her after-school religion class, and I was home cooking. I thought it strange that John walked into the house with lots of food from McDonald's, knowing that I was making dinner.

"They forced me to stop and get them food," he said.

John sat down on the couch and watched television for a few minutes; then he went to bed. I was so worn out emotionally that I had forgotten to pick up Kristen from her after school religion class, and was about 45 minutes late. I realized that I hadn't even called Gail, to say that I wouldn't be there to help out with the class.

I thought back to what had happened a few days before. Father McLaughlin was giving a sermon at Mass. The four kids, ages 9 through 16, were all lined up in the pew. We looked like such a nice, happy family.

During the sermon, Father used the analogy of a little green turtle trying to climb out of a glass fish bowl. I thought back to the little green turtles we had bought at Grant's Five-and-Dime when we were kids, and the plastic bowl with the little plastic palm tree in the middle.

"It keeps sliding down. There's no way out," said the priest.

I don't remember what he was talking about, but I clearly remember John's response. He leaned over towards me and mouthed the words, "That's me. There's no way out."

I had talked to the priest a couple of weeks before. "Father, my husband is losing his job and he's very stressed out. Can you talk to him?"

He told me to have John call him. John wasn't up for that. I don't think John even heard that suggestion. John's hopelessness was alarming me.

I saw John's sister in the back of the church. "Johnny is really in a bad way." She said, "Come over to our house right now." She made a nice meal for us, roast beef, asparagus, and a delicious dessert. She reassured John that he would be all right, reminding him that we all go through ups and downs.

I felt like he was ruining everything because he was so stressed out. The anxiety medication and the sleep medicine were not working, and his moods were constantly fluctuating.

One night, I got so burned out that I lashed out and shouted, "You're driving me crazy. I feel like killing myself!" The whole or-deal had become overwhelming.

I didn't really mean it; I didn't truly feel like that. I don't even know where the words came from. I just said the most shocking thing I could think of, not on purpose, the words just fell from my mouth. Perhaps, unconsciously, it was to jolt him into listening to me.

I knew that things were really bad, because there was no reaction at all on John's part, when I said this.

He never actually said anything about killing himself, but I remembered having had a fleeting thought of him standing near a bridge on his way to work. One morning, he just looked so weak. He was standing in our bedroom, wearing the same burgundy striped shirt that he had worn the day before. I remember exactly where he was standing, right by the telephone in our bedroom. I was over on the other side of the room , near the bed. There was just something about his look that day, that made me a little fearful.

For a guy, who was a "clothes horse" and an impeccable dresser, this was a bad sign. He always wore a classy gold tie bar, snazzy cufflinks and the finest of suits with crisp, starched shirts. A camel hair overcoat always finished his impeccable outfit. I felt that he was fading.

April 28, 1999

It was sunny, picture-perfect. It was bright. It was warm. It was a beautiful Wednesday morning. I heard John's voice as I awoke from a sound sleep. "Trish, there's something wrong with me. I just tried to kill myself. I was driving around."

"John, where did you go," I asked, alarmed, prickled with fear. "I went to the bridge, but I couldn't do it," he answered.

It was all starting to feel like a nightmare. We spent a beautiful April morning sitting in the emergency room. My husband had told me a few hours earlier that he'd gone to a bridge to jump, but couldn't do it—then breathed in carbon monoxide from the car.

Am I really sitting in a psychiatric crisis center? I wondered. *My husband should be at work right now, and I should be making beds and walking the dog.*

It was a weekday. What happened to my routine?

A psychiatric worker was gathering John's intake information, and I was waiting outside the room.

"Mrs. Gallagher, we're now taking your husband in for an examination to check his stomach for carbon monoxide residue or damage."

A short time later, John joined me on the orange vinyl chairs. I asked if we could go to the cafeteria. John was like a zombie. He ordered a pasta dish but didn't even touch it.

On the elevator ride back to the waiting room, I ran into an acquaintance from my children's school. She said, "Hi, what are you doing here?" I said I was visiting a relative.

At the crisis center, another psychiatric clerk talked to John privately, then asked me to come in. He said that John had almost all of the classic signs of depression. Next to each indicator on his list of signs, he had placed a check: 1) feelings of sadness;

depressed mood/and or irritability, 2) loss of interest in activities/hobbies, 3) changes in weight or appetite, 4) sleeping too much; not sleeping at all, 5) feelings of guilt, hopelessness or worthlessness, and 6) inability to concentrate or remember things; to make decisions.

He asked John if he was planning to harm himself. John said, "No."

I took the clerk aside, and questioned his asking John such a question. "Wouldn't that be putting ideas into his head?" I asked.

They said that they were waiting for a room. We sat waiting there for what seemed like an eternity.

The observation sheet said:

Number of observation hours: 10 hours/40 minutes.

Diagnosis: Major Depression.

Ten hours and 40 minutes is a long time for a patient and his wife to sit on orange vinyl chairs in a hospital waiting room!

We were told that outpatient treatment might be recommended after an evaluation by a psychiatrist in the morning.

I was outraged. My thoughts were racing. *How can you even consider outpatient treatment? For a man who hasn't slept in four months, has gone down to $159^3/4$ pounds, and just tried to kill himself?"*

I pleaded with the clerk:

"I just told you he was driving around at 6 a.m. this morning, when I didn't even know he was out of the house. He breathed in carbon monoxide. He said he was thinking of jumping from a bridge. Please don't send him home. I can't watch him around the clock. I can't do anything to help him myself."

We waited. We sat all day and all night until they agreed at 10 p.m. to give him a bed in the psychiatric ward.

In the intake report, they had called it "suicide ideation," because he hadn't taken the carbon monoxide in an enclosed area. He had pulled to the side of the road and breathed the exhaust from his car. This was "ideation."

But, finally, it was acknowledged in the Emergency report that he needed to be hospitalized.

Patient made a serious suicide attempt on 4/28/99 by sniffing carbon monoxide exhaust fumes. Patient is a danger to himself and needs in-patient hospitalization for safety of self.

I drove home extremely shaken. I felt ignored for those many hours, sitting and waiting for the elusive bed. We had watched television, while sitting there. Dr. Phil was a guest on the Oprah Show. He was talking about dieting. John didn't want to watch it. He told me to tell the worker that he had an eating disorder. Eating disorder, what did he mean by that?

The report continued:

Patient's wife verbalized that in the recent past, John has been obsessed with eating enough and concerned he was getting too thin. Wife identifies this preoccupation as a source of stress for patient.

I thought back to the bags of food John bought at the grocery store—and never ate. He was losing weight rapidly, while also bringing home food—food that got wasted in the refrigerator.

While in the waiting room, I called the therapist that John had seen the week before. I had seen her afterwards, myself. She asked me to call her when I got home. I called her about 11 p.m., and told her that they had admitted John for the night, and that he would be seen by the psychiatrist in the morning. We talked about the outpatient treatment plan that they had discussed while we were waiting.

"He really is determined to kill himself," the therapist said to me. It sounded so bizarre to me. Yet, I was certain that he was beyond outpatient treatment; I told her so. She concurred, and suggested that I call another psychiatric facility to see if an inpatient bed was available for the next day.

Robin and Katelyn were in their bedrooms. I didn't know that they were listening on the telephone extension while I spoke to the therapist.

"Mom, you didn't tell us that Dad tried to commit suicide," they cried in horror. I had told the kids that their father had gone into the hospital that morning, and that they were keeping him overnight because he had pains.

The next morning, following a consultation John had with a staff psychiatrist, the social worker called me with the recommendation that he go home and come back a few days later for their day program. The hospital social worker was very kind, and explained that there were just a few people in the day program. She assured me that John would get good care.

"I need to think about that. I'll call you back," I said.

I prayed, and called the therapist again, asking, "Should he be in the day program, or go somewhere else for inpatient treatment?"

My husband was emotionally and physically drained. I called the social worker that I had spoken to during our long wait the day before. During that conversation, we had talked about the possibility of sending John to another hospital. Now, on the phone, she told me that she had called the other hospital and that there was no bed available until the next day.

The choice was this: I could either agree to their day program recommendation, which would not begin for a few more days, or go to the other facility, the following morning. Both choices meant that I had to take him home.

I thought of how we had sat in the waiting room the day before, practically ignored, until 10 p.m. There had been little nurturing, kindness, medicine, or therapy. It seemed like apathy to me.

It was also an insurance matter. The insurance provider had approved a 24-hour observation, and that's what they were doing: simply observing him. To me, it seemed like simply ignoring him—and me.

When I got back to the hospital in the morning, I found that he was traumatized from the overnight stay in the psychiatric ward.

"They wouldn't let me have my shoelaces, and I had to ask for a razor blade to shave. I was so afraid of the other patient in my room. He was crazy, so they moved me to another room. I'm never going to a place like that again. It's like an insane asylum. It was scary."

I decided to have him discharged, and to admit him to the other hospital the following morning. As we left the hospital, with a prescription for Paxil, I felt nervous. I didn't want to go back to our house. I drove to Tyler Park where we had spent many happy hours sitting by the creek. He didn't seem to be "with it." I had to go to the rest room, but I was afraid to leave him. I thought, *What if he gets into the van and drives away? What if he throws himself into the water?* He repeated that he never wanted to go back to that hospital for fear he would be cut off from everybody.

I was on high alert. I didn't know what to expect anymore. The John I had been married to for close to 22 years was not acting like himself, the "real John." It seemed like our lives had gone haywire.

I asked him directly, "John, why would you do that to us? Try to kill yourself? I would never do that to you."

His face was totally blank. It was as if he had not heard a word I said.

Going to the park hadn't worked. *Where can we go?* I asked myself. *Where can we go?*

I drove to a monastery and went into the church—a church, where I had been going daily for about a year, praying for a job for John, a solution to his medical problems, and peace for the family.

This didn't work. When we got there, he said, "Take me back to the hospital. I can't cope." I turned the car around and started to drive home. I stopped the car and parked in a convenience store parking lot. We sat in the car for a few minutes, and then I thought of a place that he normally loved to go—the Olive Garden. So I drove there. We went inside, and ordered food. But he didn't touch his food. When we left, we passed The Sport's Authority, and his face lit up with excitement. A new man was emerging, one I had not seen in months.

"That's where I would love to work," he said.

By the time we arrived home, his total demeanor had changed. It was euphoric. "Trish, I feel better. I'm back to myself. I'm going to write a book about this. I'm back to myself." I hadn't seen "this John" in many months. Of course, I didn't quite believe this was real. *I know drugs are good but how could all of this fear really go away after just one Paxil at the hospital this morning?*, I wondered.

That day, he did a special activity with each of the kids. He took Ryan to collect golf balls from a field, Katelyn to get water ice, Kristen to the library, and Robin to apply for a job at Super Fresh. I breathed a sigh of temporary relief, and lay down to rest. Everyone was out of the house, and I tried to process the craziness of the past twenty-four hours.

A neighbor came over, concerned, "I hear John was in the hospital. Is he all right?" he asked.

I lied. "Yeah, he's fine." I said. "He just went in for a test." Around dusk, John returned and then went to the store. I wor

ried. *Is that where he's really going?* I thought.

Meanwhile, Robin, age 16, said she was going for a run. I didn't want her to go. It was dark and dangerous. She left anyway. I put my concerns for her on the back burner, and went to the store to check on John.

He wasn't in the supermarket, but the neighbor that I had tried to avoid was. There was also a chatty lady from my church. I ran from the store and looked for John's car. My mind raced as I wondered where he was. Maybe he went to a bridge. . . . I imagined him slumped over the front seat of his car, with a gunshot wound.

Now where? I asked myself. *Where could he be?* I ran into the drug store and saw him in the next aisle. I stood there watching him. My mind was racing; I was hyper-vigilant. *Is he buying those pills to overdose? Those razor blades to do himself harm?*

He could be just buying those razor blades for his personal shaving needs, I told myself; I shouldn't overreact. If he saw me standing here, it might make things worse. So I left. But I was on high alert about anything that I thought might cause harm. I drove home with fear in my heart.

Robin still wasn't home from her jog. I was worried about both of them. Much later, I found out that he had gone to the drugstore to pick up his prescription for Paxil. It was a new prescription, pre-scribed by the discharge psychiatrist that morning at the hospital. John had never taken an anti-depressant before. And Robin arrived home safely.

We both fell asleep exhausted. At around 4:00 a.m., I awoke from a deep sleep, to the sound of John pacing in our bedroom. Then, interspersed with the pacing, I heard retching sounds from the bathroom, like he was trying to cough something up.

I thought of the Paxil, and got up and gave him one. Then I went back to bed, exhausted beyond belief. It sounded like he was gagging. I just lay there, monitoring everything, mainly listening to see if he would leave the bedroom. I was waiting to see if he was going to walk downstairs, or out the door, or—to the garage.

He came back to bed and we fell asleep. I tried to put his arm around me, as he kept it every night before, but his arm went limp. It was yet another night of John sweating and shaking. It was just another sign that the "real John" that I had known and loved so much was not there.

On April 30th, around 7a.m., I went over to his side of the bed to tell him that I was going to take our fourteen-year-old daughter, Katelyn, to choral practice. He appeared dead. His face was ashen, his eyes fixed wide open, like a scared deer, shocked by headlights.

He did not respond to my screams, "John! John!" My first thought was that he had worried himself into a heart attack, and then I thought of the bottle of Paxil. I screamed to my children, "Call 911! Daddy's dead!"

I frantically called Diana and Nancy, two of my neighbors, and said, "John's dead." Kristen, age 11, ran next door for help. Within minutes, Diana, an ER nurse, rolled him on the floor to jolt him out of his comatose state. His eyes flickered. He was alive.

His first words were "I took carbon monoxide. I don't have a brain." Diana assured him, "John, that can't happen. You still have a brain." He was confused. He had taken carbon monoxide two days before.

Within minutes, as I stood there in my peach chenille bathrobe, our house filled up with paramedics, police and strangers. Neighbors were cuddling my children downstairs. The dog was jumping on everyone. The mood was somber. It was surreal.

It was a beautiful spring day. We were a "normal" family. How could all this be happening to us?

We stood him up and tried to put his pants and shoes on, for his trip to the hospital. He didn't seem to understand how to do it himself. With help, he walked to the ambulance, and they laid him in the back. I said to the officer, "He was in the hospital on Wednesday because he took carbon monoxide."

The man's response startled me: "Do you have any firearms in the house? If so, now's the time to remove them."

Katelyn rode in the front seat of the ambulance, while I changed from my bathrobe, called my parents and comforted Ryan and Kristen. I then took the two children to Nancy's house, so my parents could pick them up and drive them to school. Robin, who was in 11th grade, was on her way to school, unaware that all of this was happening. I jumped in my van and went to the ER to catch up with the ambulance. I remember passing my parents as they were going to Nancy's house.

I don't know how the children even focused that day, after having such a shock and witnessing such a commotion in the morning. Of course, the teachers could have had no idea what these two little kids had experienced only an hour before.

It was Friday, April 30th. We were en route, separately, heading back to the same hospital that had kept him overnight on Wednesday, April 28th, and discharged him Thursday morning, April 29th, with a recommendation to come back for the day program.

As he waited, on the bed, in the ER, I could tell he was not thinking clearly. He said, "Trish, they are not going to kill me, are they?" I went up to the hospital crisis worker and told him each time, I heard or thought of something that was critical for them to know. The worker responded, "Mrs. Gallagher, you are inundating us with information." I went up to the doctor at the desk and asked, "Doctor, what happened to him this morning? Why was he unconscious in bed?" In a detached and slightly irritated tone, he responded, "First you have to get his blood pressure under control and then his mental illness."

I went home for a few hours, to regroup, take a shower and get dressed in a decent outfit. I dabbed on some perfume, put on an attractive burlap dress, with a scarf and artfully applied my make-up. I wanted to redeem myself because of the way I looked, when I followed the ambulance in the morning. I wanted people to know that we were a "normal family' and that we had it together. I wanted John to see me looking attractive and happy. Maybe that would make him feel better. I wasn't used to seeing John so blue.

My immediate thought was of how insensitive he was and then I thought, mental illness…he must have us mixed up with some other family. He must be thinking of another patient. We are a normal family, no mental illness here!

A few hours later, John was placed on the cardiac floor, to treat his high blood pressure. Supposedly, he did not meet the criteria for admission for psychiatric care. He had apparently convinced the mental health crisis worker that he was not suicidal.

Patient seems anxious. Patient expressed no suicide ideation. Patient was evaluated by mental health crisis worker, and deemed inappropriate for psychiatric admission. Will admit for BP (blood pressure) and further evaluation

Evaluated yesterday at this hospital for suicide attempt, cleared by psychiatrist for outpatient partial program.

ER arranging for a medical bed – 3 medical.

I stood by the bed, and showed him a photo album of the kids, trying to cheer him up. Something that I thought would distract him from his anxiety.

He said, "I can't look at that. It reminds me of when I used to be happy."

Months later he told me he had been thinking, "Everything looks so good—you, the kids, me. Everything looks so perfect, and I have so many imperfections."

He asked me to call my mother to bring him some clothes. I left the room to use the phone in the nurse's station.

As I walked back to his room, I heard someone scream, "**Was there a patient in room 318? Someone just jumped out that window!**"

I ran. The window was open. I looked down to a cement walk-way—and saw him lying face up.

I screamed, "**My husband jumped out the window!**"

Someone yelled, "**Call 911!**"

The nurse's report described the sequence of events:

I had four interactions with the patient. At 7:00 he was admitted to the floor and oriented to his room. He was ambulatory, pleasant, smiled and made eye contact. The second time, Mr. Gallagher came to the desk and asked for a newspaper or magazine. I walked into the hallway to show him the visitor's lounge. Shortly afterwards, I returned to his room to see if he had found anything. He had found magazines and was sitting in a chair next to his bed, reading. The third time, he again came to the desk requesting water. I walked with him to the pantry, showed him where cups and crackers were, and showed him where to find beverages. He smiled, thanked me and made eye contact. He walked back to his room. Lastly I went to question him on his emergency contact person's name and phone number, and to find out which of his prescription meds he had taken. At this time, I sat on his bed while he was in the chair next to me. He denied taking his prescribed Paxil and Mavik. His wife came in to visit. I asked who his visitor was, and he introduced her as his wife. I got up to let her sit next to him, and left the room. This was approximately 7:15 p.m. At 7:30, his wife came screaming out into the hallway and stated that her husband had "jumped out the window." Upon arrival at the patient's room, the window was found open. 911 was called.

The doctor's notes read:

Patient apparently jumped out of his bedroom (Room 318) window about 7:30 p.m. Call placed to 911 for ambulance, immediately. Patient found down on concrete in front of hospital. Patient was conscious (groaned to verbal stimulus), with adequate pulse and respirations. Airway patent and stable. Bilateral femoral fx apparent. Oxygen administered and IV fluids begun, with assistance of hospital staff. Police and ambulance arrived (approx. 5 minutes), assisted ambulance crew in patient stabilization.

I waited frantically to see him, but a nurse said, "I'm sorry, you can't. They're working on him." She was kind, and asked,

"Do you want to pray?" We said the Lord's Prayer together. I went outside and sat on a bench. One of the ER doctors sat next to me, and very somberly apologized and said, "I am so sorry. I thought I was do-ing the right thing."

I cried. "I told you he was going to hurt himself!"

I didn't know if John was alive. They asked me what faith I was, and I said Catholic. I was then seated in a room with a priest and some of the hospital staff. My father, brother-in-law, and sister-in-law came and sat in the room with us. Then we all went to the trauma center, located about 15 minutes away. Outside, it was a beautiful, warm April evening.

I thought of the line from the nursery rhyme: "Along came a spider and sat down beside her and frightened Miss Muffet away." The spider was depression: big, black, scary. It had literally

frightened John away—almost permanently.

He had been running on empty emotionally for a prolonged period, tangled in a web of despair. The depression had stolen his sense of peace, happiness and self-esteem. And now, it seemed to be grabbing me, too.

I thought of the way he had been chewing his lip anxiously the past few weeks. He wasn't doing his usual 50 push-ups on the bedroom floor.

Why didn't I notice this as a sign of foreboding? Yes, that's how I felt: all tangled up and frightened.

I needed to talk to somebody about how I felt about my husband's suicide attempt.

We agreed to tell everybody that he had fallen down the steps, or that he was in an accident. I remember saying to the psychiatrist, " What are we going to tell everybody. John won't want anybody to know." He said, "Well, this kind of story is *juicy.*"

He was in the hospital for five weeks. When he was first treated in the ER, he was in danger of a life-threatening infection from the chips of shattered bones. As strange as this sounds, I thought *where could John go until he recovers?* I thought of renting a hotel room in a town 15 minutes away or asking the nuns if he could stay in the monastery. I guess my thought process was that we have to *hide* this so nobody would ask us questions.

He was seriously injured, yet he couldn't understand why I needed to talk about it—he just wanted to forget it ever happened.

Yes, he was the one who had been in so much emotional pain for the thirteen months prior to jumping, and he was the one who was suffering with so much physical pain now. But I, too, had suffered. We all had suffered, John, me and the four children.

And, now, at this moment, there was a strange sense of relief. He is safe, he is in a hospital. We don't have to worry about him. I had experienced total shock—looking down from the third floor hospital window at my husband's lifeless body laying on the ground.

I started to think that I didn't know him at all.

The next day, at home, I went from room to room, closet to closet, and box to box, and threw away everything related to his job. He blamed the company for his stress, and I wanted every reminder of that out of our house.

I got out all of our bills and personal papers—mortgage documents, insurance documents—and put them in an organized file. I paid all of the bills. I was in a frenzied state of mind, trying to process all that had happened in the last three days.

As crazy, as it sounds, I needed to get organized. I cleaned out my closet, boxed things for the Goodwill and got all of our affairs in order. In case he did it again and died, I would be prepared.

Then, I searched all of his drawers and attaché case for any hint of a reason to attempt suicide. *Was he having an affair? Had he had a baby with someone else? What shame or circumstance would cause him to hurt his kids and me in this way? Wasn't there something dreadful going on in my husband's life that he couldn't tell me?*

I found nothing.

I did find other, more mundane things, however. There was a notebook filled with information about a comprehensive job search plan that was unsuccessful. Lists of interview dates. The outcome of each meeting. A 12-point list of things that were stressing him out. (I was on that list.)

I found several TO DO lists written neatly on his detailed "list-maker", scads of loose leaf paper:

get RX for Restoril, work out, Doctor G. at 8:30, Ryan baseball practice, Business Unit Meeting, Doctor C. Wednesday at 10:00., return library books, clean the shower

And then, a list of employment agencies, with contact names penciled in on the margin, with squiggly lines. And then a list of more things to do:

work out a deal with work, learn new computer programs, withdraw stock options to cover bills, do taxes, do spreadsheet analysis, analyze capital for intercompany profit, buy ENSURE, get Meritine, Sustecal, think of new way to get to work without bumper-to-bumper traffic

I stumbled upon more of his efforts to provide for the family. Ideas for home businesses:

physical therapy and recreational activities for the elderly; fixing air conditioners and heat pumps; renting machines from Shop'n Bag to clean carpets; painting; learning guitar and then teaching it; cleaning houses; helping Kristen sell Beanie Babies; a T-shirt shop; making cakes, popcorn, pretzels and cookies to sell.

There were scads of papers, with columns drawn with blue ball-point pen—his "what-if" scenarios:

WORST—I lose my job and get a severance package

BEST—take another job; if it doesn't work out, look for another job; talk to Human Resources and ask how much longer I have to find another job

DO NOTHING - still have to do my job, still have to look for a job, department going away, will lose job, talk to boss and tell her not happy; she is calling the shots

My husband was meticulous about things—always a neat wallet, a tidy garage, and bureau drawers in perfect order. He never took off an article of clothing without folding it neatly and putting it back in his drawer. His closets were arranged in perfect order, with suits, shirts, belts and ties arranged like an exclusive men's clothier.

And there was another thing he was meticulous about—our children's safety. He always insisted on seatbelts. He worried about them going too far out in the ocean, or falling off of the railing of the boardwalk. He would constantly say, "Trish, watch her; she's too close to the railing." He would never choose a second floor rental property at the shore.

He was not a risk taker, and was certainly not impulsive. He liked to plan every detail of everything—a picnic, a job search, a vacation. Lists were made and lists were followed. I liked that about him. Nothing last-minute. It worked for us.

He was a hard worker, and rarely took a day off from work unless he was really sick. He was conscientious.

As I searched his notes, my mind wandered to stories I had read in the news about people who had hurt their families while under psychiatric care. I wondered, *Would we be safe when he came home?*

I went to the hospital twice daily to visit him and then, when he came home, I took care of him. It was overwhelming. Hot summer weather, plus four active children, picking up prescriptions, making doctor's appointments, and watching him struggle to walk. It was awful.

A few people knew the truth about what happened, but we limited ourselves to only telling a few trusted friends and relatives. Although they were a good source of support, I wanted to talk. I needed to share my innermost fears with someone else.

Several weeks after the accident, I was giving a seminar at a major university, when I noticed the time: 7:27 PM. I couldn't contain myself. It triggered the memory of John jumping at 7:27 PM on a Friday night a few weeks earlier. I lost my train of thought, and blurted out my woes to the students. I went off on a totally inappropriate tangent about my own personal tragedy, asking the group to please not repeat it, because two of my children did not even know.

Another day, I went to pick up family photos at Wal-Mart, and became argumentative with the young sales clerk who waited on me. I raised my voice, and fussed with her over a coupon offer. I was totally out of line. Then, when the store's greeter asked about my husband in the wheelchair, I told her that he had jumped out of a window—then asked her to swear that she wouldn't tell anyone.

I felt disloyal to my husband when I shared our business. I told about thirty people: people I knew in towns far from where we lived, the lady in Wal-Mart, the people in the class, strangers in New York City.

We had not told his father and our good neighbors and friends. I was afraid that the word would get out and get back to my husband—or that my nine-year-old son would find out the truth. I didn't want people saying, "Why did your dad jump out a window?" or spreading rumors: "Oh, he's the guy that tried to commit suicide." I didn't want gossip.

I knew that I had been compassionate throughout the past year—that I had tried to be supportive and to take care of all of the things he used to do. I didn't mind that he slept a lot, even though I knew that it wasn't normal. Only once, in the privacy of our bedroom, did I ask him, "How could you do this to us?" Even when I did that, I wasn't really mad at him. I knew how much pain he was in. Most of the time, I tried to stay upbeat.

Looking back, I realize that I couldn't have known how much pain he was in. I had never had depression. I could never even begin to understand.

Whose fault was all of this, anyway? There were times when I wanted to cast blame. Why, for example, didn't the primary doctor call me to tell me John needed psychiatric help? Why didn't the doctors and the staff at the hospital listen to my pleas? Why wouldn't the insurance company approve the proper care that John required?

Shortly after John's fall, however, while rummaging through his wallet and briefcase, I found two referrals from his primary doctor for him to get psychiatric care, and one for biofeedback therapy.

The truth was that John had not pursued those suggestions. He was so immersed in his pain that he was not capable of following through. He had just run out of emotional steam to figure things out on his own and I didn't know a thing about the referrals, or depression.

Some people tried to be helpful, giving unsolicited advice. Although I am sure that their intentions were good, they made me uneasy.

Others scared me. Two people whose loved ones had succeeded in killing themselves told me that John would do it again—and succeed. I didn't want to believe this.

After he was home for about six months, he was able to drive. I was nervous about that. I didn't think he had adequate control of his leg muscles. When he got upset or went to bed for the day, I worried. When he left the house, and looked like he was feeling a little blue, I followed him. I didn't want him to think I didn't trust him, but I was scared. We had kids to raise together, and I didn't want to miss a signal that he was depressed again.

I also hated to ask him if he had taken his medicine, because I knew that it was his responsibility—but if he forgot, we would be the ones living without him. Sometimes one of the kids would say,

"Mom, I think you better follow him. I don't think he's really going to the grocery store."

The medicine he took made him tired. On some occasions, this caused alarm. Once, he went to return a few library books and hadn't returned after a few hours. In my mind's eye, I pictured a bridge. I didn't know whether to call the police, or ask family members to help me look for him. As it turned out, he had fallen asleep in the parking lot.

I hoped that life would soon get back to normal. I didn't want John's reputation tarnished. He had coached our kids' sports teams for several years, and I didn't want his illness to interfere or prevent him from doing this. I feared that people would say: "I don't want my kids driving with him. That guy's unstable."

And yet, I might have reacted that way myself if I were watching the situation unfold in someone else's life.

I needed a friend who had been through this. I wanted to know what was going on.

Would it get better? Why was I feeling the way I was? Would he ever heal from the physical and psychological fallout of a major depression? Would he always need antidepressants? Would we ever snuggle together and laugh and take drives together, like in the past?

I cried for the residual damage to our family and our marriage—and for his pain. I cried for the knowledge of his future operations, and for the 13-inch scars on his legs and hip. I also cried for our emotional scars, scars wrought by the confusion and sadness we both carried.

One day, I would be sympathetic about the depression he had suffered, and the next I would be mad at him for all of the problems he was causing the kids and me. He never seemed sorry or apologetic for our pain. His pain was so great, he did not seem able to see ours.

I went to a therapist, attended support group meetings, and found comfort talking to my older children. Yet I felt alone with the family secret.

Depression was a foreign word to our family. Suicide attempts happened to other families, with problems, right? Not to a "normal" family, I thought. I had a lot to learn. My journey had just begun. Why hadn't I known about all of the classic symptoms of depression—anger, anxiety, tension, worrying, fatigue, headaches, hypertension, indigestion and insomnia? Why hadn't I known how dangerous these symptoms were?

I also had ambivalent feelings. "Oh, it must be so hard for you to have John in the hospital," a neighbor said. In actuality, I felt a little guilty for thinking how nice it was.

The time prior to the suicide attempt was so chaotic for all of us. John had the depression, and we had the fallout. We had been completely centered on trying to cheer John up and most of the time, we weren't successful. He was still so down and we couldn't figure out what was going on. It had been going on for almost a year. John had changed. I didn't even think of depression. That word was not even in our family lexicon.

Yet we wanted "normal" again. I didn't feel like he was my husband anymore. He had no energy, no interest in activities. He was irritable with the kids, and didn't even want to play his guitar. Something was terribly wrong. We walked on eggshells around him.

So, while he was in the hospital, it was nice. Neighbors brought covered dish meals, and did things to cheer us up. Our focus was on living again, not just on trying to survive. His absence gave us the respite we needed. The heaviness of day-to-day worry had lifted.

Looking back, I wish that the whole experience had not been that of a secret we had to cover up. Depression, I now realize, is a treatable illness that can be helped with the right diagnosis, therapy, and medication. It is nothing to be ashamed of.

My message to readers is to not overlook the power that stress exerts on the human mind. My husband seemed like the kind of guy who had everything to live for. Yet the pressure of an impending layoff was a situational trigger for serious depression. We all need to pay attention to the way stress affects us and our loved ones.

I still have many unanswered questions:

Did the depression cause him to exaggerate the danger he was in at work?

Was he really losing his job or did the depression make him think he was?

When and why did he lose the power to combat the dark cloud he was under?

What triggered such an act against himself?

There were many subtle warnings, but they had eluded me. Yet we beat the odds. John survived, miraculously. He was given

a second chance. I pray now that we can find the meaning in this, and use our experience to help others.

God saved his life. I am looking for answers in His mysterious ways. I am looking for the hand of God to direct us.

Right before my husband went in for a second operation, my mother gave him a card that read:

I said to the man that stood at the gate, 'Give me a light that I may tread safely into the unknown.' And he said, 'Go out into the darkness and put thine hand into the hand of God. This will be to thee better than a light and safer than a known way.'

The experience we have had reiterates this simple advice. My entire family has suffered, but like the mythical phoenix rising from the ashes—we are coming back again, with a life that is new. And yet, we know that it is not a fairy tale. John's depression—and our sadness—did not miraculously disappear. But, along the way, we have learned something important about understanding and compassion and survival—and we hope that what we have learned can help others to "tread safely into the unknown."

Dear Trisha,

I printed the entire book so I could read it thoroughly. I was especially touched by Katelyn's story. She will never know of course, but I related far more than I would like to. The information was excellent but I can only assume the story was all about John. That being said, it was courageous and helpful to others. However, as I was so involved with you at the time, the aspect I believe would have helped families the most would have been the help you sought for yourself. I know it wasn't easy mainly because when you saw me, I was very straight forward, insisting you help yourself. If my honesty hurt you, I am sorry for that. Your description of yourself of course was right on target right down to the denial and fear, but not what you had to look at during therapy. I don't know the other therapists of whom you speak. I only know you were one of my toughest challenges running, running, running. You would not allow me to work with your grief and loss which in my opinion were massive pain centered. I don't think you ever recognized your own pain in its intensity, only John's. Remember the "moving forward focus group" that you attended? The ladies in the group tried hard to help but became frustrated with you as it was all about John. I think they played a role in helping you deal with what was going on. I am sure there were many others you have asked to read a draft of your book but most of those people were not with you during your agony. You didn't mention divorce I believe your children did. By the way, they are totally remarkable. How are things today? The last time we met, you were separated again. What happened then? Are you still living with your mother? Where are your children? Is Katelyn still in Ireland? Please bring me up to date. I truly hope life is beginning to look brighter for you.

Dr. Yvonne Kaye
www.yvonnekaye.com

Robin's Story

After nine years and all of the therapy I have been through, this is the only time I have actually been forced to go back and relive what happened to my dad, and to realize how much it affected me. Not only have I been in denial, but I have also tried very hard to suppress my feelings and act like it never happened. I didn't tell anyone the truth, for fear they would judge me or my family.

The hardest part was that, ever since we were little, our dad always wanted us to behave. I had to be the responsible one, to set the example for my siblings. Either way, I never wanted to let him down or embarrass him in any way.

My father would strive to be fair; he never had a favorite, and treated us all equally. Even though we would ask him to pick one, he would say that he loved us all the same.

My dad was the type of father who coached our basketball teams, helped us with our homework, made us pancakes for breakfast and cooked spaghetti for dinner.

He always wanted to do things the right way; he was a perfectionist. His dresser was always neat, his car was always clean, he always dressed perfectly—like he had it all together.

However, what we didn't know was that he had been suffering from depression. We knew that his mother died when he was nine years old, but what we didn't know was how much her death affected him and the fact that depression was in our family genes.

With all of that being said, I would like to go back to my junior year in high school. Like any teenager, I was so wrapped up in what I was doing that I neglected to see what was going on with my dad. I remember him being irritable and not attending family functions. My mom would get upset and my dad would just sleep more. I remember him taking off from work, and going to see doctors because of his headaches and high blood pressure.

In the weeks before my dad's "accident," it felt as if we were walking on eggshells around both my mom and dad. Our mom would tell us that our dad was very sick, for us to try and keep the house clean, but we didn't believe her. We thought that she was just frustrated with my dad and wanted us to clean the house.

On April 30, 1999, we quickly realized that my mom wasn't lying, and that her biggest fear had actually come true. My dad tried to take his life by jumping out of a three-story hospital building. The night of the so-called accident, my sister Katelyn and I were out with one of our friends. I am not sure of how my neighbor found us, but she quickly brought us to the hospital. I remember her not saying much to us and how I nervously tried to make conversation with her.

As soon as we got to the hospital, our mother's father, my grand-father, was waiting outside of the trauma emergency doors. He was crying, and that is when I didn't know if my father was dead or alive. He brought us into the chapel waiting room; my aunt and uncle were there. Then I saw my mom. She was sitting down, and looked up at me and said, "Daddy jumped out of the window."

I am not sure of how much of that I was able to process, but Katelyn and I just held each other and walked out of the room. I remember that we went to the vending machines and were in complete shock. I recall being grateful that I had her there with me. We spent the night at the hospital, waiting for my dad's surgery to be over. I think it was either that night or the night after that we all slept in my parents' bed with my mom, just holding each other and praying that my dad would be okay.

After that night, it all seems a blur to me. I can remember being in the psychiatric ward a couple of times, thinking that everyone in there was so crazy. I didn't think my dad belonged there. I can still visualize my dad returning home—with his hospital bed in our living room, and a male nurse from Abington Homecare beside him, someone who resembled Elvis.

Our neighbors were very supportive, and my mom was strong. She really held it all together for us. I believe this happened during my junior year in high school, but I don't remember our family really falling apart until my freshman year in college. I know that I definitely rebelled as a freshman. I had been a really good student in high school, but was upset that I didn't go away for college and that my parents gave me a curfew.

After my grandfather died, I decided to live with my maternal grandmother. I said it was to help her, but what I really wanted was some stability in my life. Even though I loved my family, I just needed to get away from them, and I know now that this really hurt my mom.

Now that I am able to look back, my mom has really been through a lot. Not only did she lose her husband, but she also lost her oldest daughter. Our relationship has always been great, but I can tell that there is something that is still keeping me at a distance. I think it is guilt that I didn't stay with my family when it was hard. I chose to go the easy route. After my parents separated and sold our house, I didn't move with my mom and siblings to the new house because I knew it would be chaotic. I also didn't want to leave my grandmother, and felt pulled. Since I have lived with her for many years, I don't feel that way anymore, but for so long I felt that something was missing in my life. I even got into a relationship for two years that was unhealthy. I expected my boyfriend to be there for me, and he couldn't fill that void either.

Even though I try to act like everything is okay in my family, I do have a tendency to get stressed out. Sometimes it is a little too much when my mom and dad want to talk about what happened. I remember a couple of years ago, that is all we ever talked about when we got together. It was so tense because we wanted to express how we were really feeling, but we didn't want to hurt anyone. We couldn't tell our parents the truth about what we were really feeling.

I never blamed my mom or dad for anything that happened. I know that my mom needed support from my dad with things, and that he wasn't there for her emotionally. When incidents like these happen, you can't blame anyone. I know that it is easy to hold other people responsible, but depression is a family problem. There are many factors that come into play. In all honesty, I do not know what my dad was thinking when he decided to jump out the window that day. We were never sure. We wanted to think that he did not do it on purpose. One of my sisters asked my mother, "Was Dad just trying to get out, because he was scared?" Although that did not really make any sense either, that was easier to fathom than my dad wanting to kill himself.

I have never asked my dad why he did it or why he thought that he was better off not living. Did he think of how it would affect us? Honestly, I don't need to hear anything from my dad. I just know that he is better now—and I am so proud of him. I would never want any family to have to deal with these issues, but as the saying goes, "What happens to you only makes you stronger." I feel that I am a much stronger person and that I can relate to other people who are suffering from similar concerns.

After this experience, I have come to realize that things happen unexpectedly, and that any time might be the last time I see my family. I guess that is why I have chosen not to dwell so much on what exactly happened to my dad; I am just grateful that he was all right.

Something I know that I got from my dad is to always do things the right way. I want to be perfect, to look like I have it all together. In retrospect, some days I feel like I am falling apart, while other days I am genuinely happy. I sometimes wonder if I am depressed or bi-polar—even manic at times. All I do know is that, whatever it is, my family is there for me no matter what. There is never a problem that we can't all fix together.

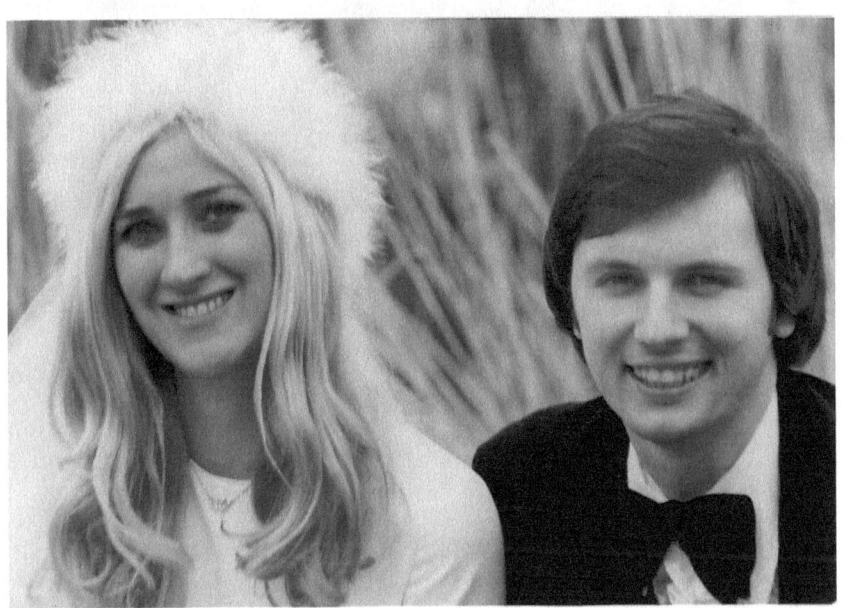

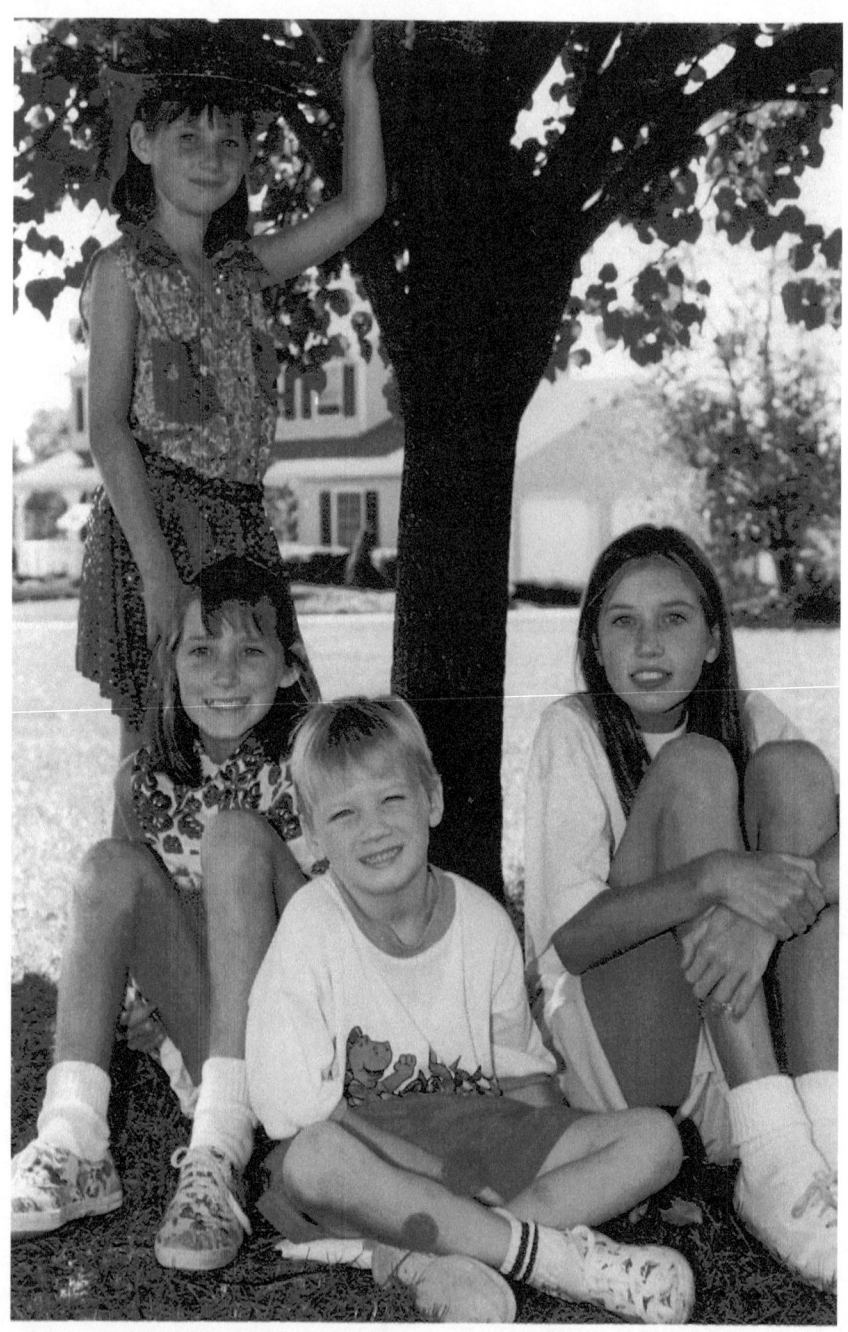

Katelyn's Story

I was about 14. I was probably about 5'2". I had a full life, or so I thought. I knew everything, or so I believed. My day would start around 7:15 a.m., when my Dad would wake me up to go to chorus practice. Actually, if I got there earlier than 7:15 a.m.— maybe 7:05 a.m.—there would be doughnuts provided by my music instructor. So, there is a possibility that I told my Dad that I had to be there earlier than 7:15. He was the one to drive me because he was leaving for work around the same time.

Every day, it was the same routine: "Katelyn, wake up! Katelyn, wake up! It's time to wake up," he would say. I just took this for granted. *Ugh*, I'd think, *I know it's time to wake up. Why won't he stop?*

But suddenly, things changed. Weeks passed, when our friendly father-daughter car rides were becoming muted. I started to feel like a burden, an errand, a task.

Maybe my dad started waking up later—or, for whatever reason—we asked a neighbor to start driving me to school. So I just thought: *Well, maybe he needs to be at work earlier. Okay, it's no big deal.* Until I realized that I wasn't just losing a ride from my dad, I also started seeing him less and less each day— sometimes not at all. He worked all the time, and I missed him.

When I did see him on the weekends, things were different; he seemed angry and annoyed.

"Why is Dad being so mean?" I'd ask my mom. "He's just sick right now," she would say.

At that time, maybe still to this day, I felt like I was the only one of my siblings that noticed the polarization of my dad's moods. It was starting to affect me like cancer. Sadness and anger were slowly taking over my innocent, happy self. I was worried sick, but I didn't understand what I was worried about. The word "depression" didn't mean anything to me. Nobody even used that word in our house. For months and years after my dad jumped, I wondered—*Why would my dad even be depressed?* He has four kids, a dog, a loving wife, and a nice house. What's his problem?

After a while, we drifted back to the old morning routine again. My father was driving me to school.

Then, one morning—a shock—I woke up myself! No alarm. No parents squawking.

There was nothing coming from my mom and dad's room. I didn't hear the usual chaotic noise of the morning rush.

I entered their room, saying "Dad, dad wake up we're going to be late, come on!"

I walked over to his side of the bed. There was no movement, no response.

"Come on!" I insisted.

This was a big day for me. On this day, I was supposed to prac-tice one more time before singing a solo in front of my whole school—in front of 1,500 or so students. *Maybe that's why I woke up on my own,* I thought. The excitement was overwhelming.

The moment I realized that my dad wasn't waking up at all, my mom and I started screaming—"**Dad's dead! He's dead! Kristen! Robin! Ryan! Daddy's dead!**"

His face was battleship colored gray, his eyes were filmy, and his body was frozen. We all panicked. My brother called 911—or tried, anyhow. He kept dialing wrong: 919, 119, 991. He couldn't function; none of us could.

Finally, the call went through and the ambulance arrived. We also called a neighbor who was a nurse.

We couldn't understand what had happened. Nothing was making sense. As they took my dad into the ambulance, they asked if anyone was coming with him. I guess my mom needed to drive her car to bring my siblings to the hospital. I said that I would go, and I sat in front of the ambulance on the passenger side.

I didn't say one word. I couldn't. I physically couldn't move my mouth. I was sweating and crying. Thoughts and emotions were racing through my mind at an incredible velocity. I remember wanting to ask the driver, "Do you think he'll be okay? Please, my dad isn't really dead, is he?" But I remained silent. I wanted to talk because I felt rude. I felt uncomfortable for not making conversation.

When we arrived at the hospital, I realized that my dad wasn't dead. They wheeled him inside and took him away to a tiny room that resembled a janitor's closet. I remember that I wasn't allowed to go with him. I had to stay in the Emergency Room until my mom arrived. Eventually, we were told that we could go into his room. He was okay but not making very much sense.

Later on that night, I spent time with my sister Robin and her friend, while my Mom was at the hospital. We went out and rented a movie and ordered pizza.

Eventually we got back to the house. Soon afterwards, the phone rang. It was my neighbor. She said she was going to be picking us up and that we needed to go to the hospital right away. Two minutes later, she was in our driveway. For nearly fifteen minutes, on the ride over, there was silence. I was frightened. Nothing was explained. I feared the worst, not knowing what to expect. My heart was beating uncontrollably.

As we pulled into the parking spot, my eyes shot directly to my grandfather standing on the sidewalk. We got out of the car and ran to him. He hugged me that moment tighter than I had felt anyone hug me before.

As I walked through the sliding doors, I saw a tiny room located diagonally from where I was standing, and there was my family sitting with the saddest faces I had ever seen. We walked in, and there was a priest or hospital chaplain trying to pacify them with his calm gestures and words.

Eventually the words poured out: "Daddy jumped out of the window three stories. He went out head first."

Immediately, I knew he was dead. *I don't have a dad anymore. Why would he do this to us?*

My heart crumbled.

My mother asked the nurse, "Is he going to be okay?" I felt sick and overwhelmed.

A nurse said, "He is alive but we don't know the extent of his injuries—if his injuries are life-threatening. He's in the operating room now."

It was uncomfortably strange to sit in a room for hours with no knowledge of whether or not my father was alive—or if I would hear his voice or feel his touch ever again. Hospital employees would pop their head in every now and then to see how we were doing. But there was no report on his status.

After a while, my sister and I left the room. We walked to the vending machine and we each bought a hot chocolate. We talked and we hugged. At that time in my life, I'm not sure that the two of us were very close. But, no other night would compare to the feeling of protection and love I received from her.

Many hours later, we were finally told that my dad was going to be okay. "His legs are mangled, but he is alive. It is going to take him a very long time to recover," they said, but— miraculously— we would be able to see him within the next few days.

I felt grateful for this, but still things were eerie. My mom, Robin, and I walked out to the parking lot hugging and holding hands. I remember getting into the car and hearing the song "In the Arms of an Angel," by Sarah McLaughlin, on the radio. I felt that it was a sign—that an angel had definitely been looking over my dad and the whole family that night.

We drove home to our empty, quiet house, and slept in my parents' bed—just the three of us—exhausted and heartbroken, but grateful and extremely thankful.

The next day, waking up to the bright sun shining through the window, I was perplexed. I thought to myself, *Wow, what a horrible dream!* Then I looked to the left and then to the right. I was lying in the middle of my parents' bed, between my sister and my mother.

It then clicked that it was reality. The next few days—maybe even the next few months—were a blur. My mom took us regularly to the hospital to see my dad.

The first day we went to the mental health ward was shocking. It was the first time I had ever witnessed people talking to themselves—I mean, having full, in-depth conversations with themselves. Some were staring at inanimate objects and giggling.

These people were completely amused, seemingly for no reason at all. Others were cursing and angry.

This whole situation might have seemed amusing in a strange way, except that my dad was "one of them." We were confused as to why they would imprison my dad in this peculiar setting, not fully accepting or understanding the seriousness of what being suicidal meant.

We wanted to keep his spirits high while he was in the hospital. When he returned home, I remember my mom telling my dad every day how her angel pin business was booming and how much money was coming in. I thought to myself, *That isn't true. Why is she trying to get his hopes up?* I was afraid he would find out the truth and become even more depressed when he came back home.

My mom wanted my dad to not worry about anything. After a month or two, my dad came home. We set up a room for him in the living room of our house. He stayed in that bed for a very long time. Physical therapists would come, and make him do exercises that would help his legs become strong again.

I don't remember much after that, except being asked a lot of questions from curious parents in the neighborhood. My friends' parents would ask how my family was doing and what exactly happened to my dad.

I remained vague. "He's fine. We're fine," I'd say.

We would tell different stories to people: "He fell down the stairs and broke his legs" or "He was in a bad car accident," hoping that that would be sufficient. But, somehow, it wasn't.

I felt like I couldn't talk to anyone about how I was feeling. I was lying to my friends, and I suddenly felt like a completely different person. I was older.

I developed an emotional armor around me to keep others away. I wanted so badly to be strong and to not make my dad feel bad about this. I never wanted him to feel sadness or pain again. I didn't want him to feel guilty for trying to leave us.

I actually felt guilty at this time, and for a long period thereafter, that maybe he had done this because of me. After all, I was always getting into trouble, wasn't I?

Everything started changing.

Even before my dad left the hospital, the subject of selling our house and moving came up. The mortgage was too high, my mom explained. If my dad wasn't going to be able to work, we would have to move to a place we could rent.

Each time my mom and I returned home from visiting the hospital, we would feel an immediate and urgent need to clean the house. I suppose this was our way of mentally cleansing ourselves. We decided that, if we cleaned, maybe we would feel better. Well, we weren't just cleaning, but obsessively picking up items in the house, taking all of the decorations down from the walls, and dragging and carrying things to put at the end of the driveway.

We lifted the couch, the tables, the beds—anything we could get our hands on—and started throwing them away. After a while, almost everything was gone. Our house looked like we were moving out or had been robbed.

We felt better for having cleared out the clutter.

A few weeks after this all happened, I was looking for a notepad in my father's top bureau drawers, when I found a handwritten list. It was a list of things he had written down that stressed him out.

I was feeling curious enough to read it. It listed: "work, money . . . KATELYN."

Me? I thought, shocked. *I am on this list!!* I recall not seeing anyone else's name on that list but my own. I can't describe the horrendous feeling that came over me at that second. It drenched me with sadness. I don't remember if I showed my mom that day or if I waited. However, I was incredulous—so very shocked and mad at myself—or at him—I didn't know which.

I was so angry that I was on that list. I think it said something about me fighting with my siblings. But, why was **I** the one to blame? They mostly initiated it, I thought to myself. Why was it so easy for them to get away with yelling at **me**?

I held on to this anger for a very long time. I was convinced that my dad didn't love me—or like me, rather. I kept this belief for maybe five or six years. I stopped trusting him.

The therapist asked me if I felt guilty at all for my dad's attempt. I would nod and indubitably say," Yes, of course, it was my fault. I saw my name on the paper."

We went to nearly a dozen therapists. As soon as we would become comfortable with one of them, our insurance would run out or the copay would increase, and we would move onto someone else. Each therapist would explain that it had nothing to do with me, my mom, or my siblings.

What my dad suffered from was a chemical imbalance, they would say, a disease. I remained firm with my initial response, though—that I was to blame—because I had made up my mind permanently. I didn't want to accept the explanations they were giving me. I felt that they gave them because they felt sorry for me.

There were some sessions where I couldn't get any words out of my mouth. I would start getting all teary. After my hour-long session had come to an end, I'd feel as if I had just sat through a funeral. I would exit the room with puffy eyes, a red face, and about ten tissues that the therapist would hand me on my way out, to use for the ride home. I tried my utmost to appear like I wasn't crying, because I knew that if I walked out and saw my mom, she would try to find out what was said, and how I was feeling. This really annoyed me.

I didn't want to talk to her, or to anyone. I was hoping that this pain would dry up—if I didn't keep picking the scab of my internal wound. My mindset, at the time, was that the whole incident was just a really bad day. The next day would come, and it would be brighter. We should focus on the present, I decided. I didn't feel that we were making the situation any better by reliving it on a daily basis.

It almost felt like a punishment that I had to talk to complete strangers and tell them how miserable I felt inside, as they would stare at me and then back at the clock.

"Okay, well that's the end of our session. I'll see you in a week," the therapist would say. *How*, I wondered, *could I feel any better with this therapy?* I would be feeling fine earlier in the day. Then they would extract my emotions, and leave me feeling weak and upset when I left.

It seemed strange to me that I was going to therapy, but my dad wasn't. My mom would get angry with him for resisting therapy. He stubbornly and repeatedly refused her attempts to help him. He didn't think he needed to go, and he became annoyed with the nagging of her voice.

Their marriage came to a halt.

My mom couldn't live anymore with his irritability, plus the burden of having to take on the role of "the only parent around." Instead of doing therapy, my dad relied on antidepressants to numb the pain.

But, after a while, he knew that he had to talk to someone—a therapist—if he didn't want to suffer anymore. Seven years ago, I would never have imagined that my life would be the way that it is right now. I guess the saying is true, that time heals all things (and that maybe therapy and/or medication helps, after all). I would never want to relive those years again. I just don't think I could cope. People love to say "It's going to be okay," but when you're in the moment and you feel the rain is never going to stop, it's hard to think that there will ever be a good day again.

My dad has healed. I would say that he is 150% better now. He is loving, inspirational, and understanding in all situations. I didn't used to feel that way about him. I know that he has become the man he has always wanted to be, and I really admire how he has overcome so many obstacles. My dad overcame his physical obstacles—healing his outer wounds by learning to walk again (even with metal rods in his legs). He has also overcome his mental obstacles of self-pity and stubbornness, in order to bring our family together. I am incredibly thankful for that.

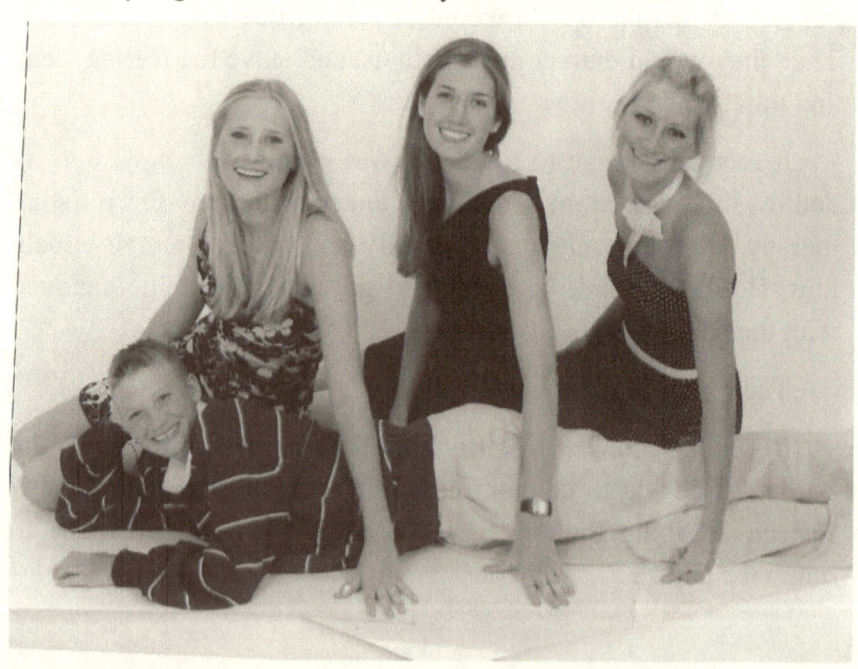

Some additional thoughts:

I was thinking long and hard about whether or not I could think of any happy or funny moments I experienced during that time. I guess I enjoyed the new "Dad" I was introduced to after the incident. My dad started on heavy medication such as antidepressants and painkillers. With crushed legs and other injuries, the doctors hoped that the medicine would bring relief both physically and emotionally. He was as "high as a kite" at times, smiling and laughing. I remember we went to dinner at Pizza Hut one night and he was laughing and trying to take pizza and soda from another person's table. This was so totally out of character for my father. My "old dad", the one before the accident, really cared about appearances. It really mattered to him how he was perceived and would never do anything that would tarnish his or the family's reputation. He cared about how he was looked at or judged ALL OF THE TIME. This is not something he would think about doing. He seemed crazier than ever, in a good way. He was childish and almost like a friend of my own age. He didn't yell at me or any of us, because I guess he didn't have the stress anymore. We watched movies together every day. His bed was downstairs now and he was always around. We weren't used to this and it was really nice to get to know my Dad.

My mom was so busy taking care of Dad, Kristen and Ryan, and working on her new business that I knew I had to take care of myself. I thought I should lay low for a while and not cause any excitement. I longed for someone to look out for me. I guess that I was confused and didn't want to stir up any trouble. I was forced to go to counseling; the counselor was the only person that I was really allowed to talk to about my problems. My mother told me later that the counselor said that I needed to get out and be with friends, that she thought I might be getting "border-line depressed."

When I was 18, I started drinking and taking pills to ease some of the pain. I was seeking the attention of my parents, but that just made us drift further apart. I couldn't deal with my anger and sadness anymore within myself or my family's house. I then moved to Ireland to be alone and on my own. Since then, I have had a lot of time to think about the past and see why I did some of the things I did in order to survive my post-traumatic stress. It has always been interesting to me how my other family members were able to see the sunny side of the street again and I was not. I wonder if they were better able to cope than I was or if it was suppression that saved them.

This is an e-mail that we received from one of the volunteers who so kindly read this manuscript before publication.

Dear Katelyn,

Thank you for writing your chapter and for your candor.

I have found myself personally touched by your story, all along. When I was 17, I found out that my father, who was just 48, was dying of cancer. He, too, needed to keep his story secret. And I, like you, am a middle child—who had many of the same perceptions and needs that you have described.

As for the question about why your siblings were more able to see the sunny side than you, I do think your guess about suppression is part of the answer. I get the sense that you felt things very deeply, in a rawer and more immediate way than the others. You perhaps suffered more because of this. But, it seems to me, that this is at least partly why the thoughts and feelings of that time are more accessible to you. Your openness throughout has been a real saving grace—

and I have total confidence that you will be able to move forward in wonderful, unimagined ways. Thanks again. I look forward to more exchanges—and, hopefully, to meeting you

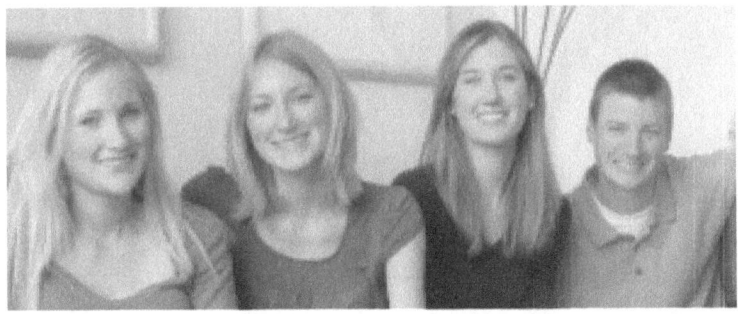

!

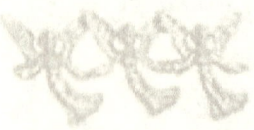

Kristen's Story

I try to go back to "that time," but memories escape me. I don't want to remember. The majority of my childhood was happy, and those few times that it wasn't just made me appreciate the other times. As I force myself to remember, I see only a few short clips. I suppose—similar to a movie—they are just brief flashes, in no particular order. But they become very vivid.

Even as I write this, I shake inside as I recall the scariest memory I have, which is probably the same as that of my brother and sisters.

It was a school day, so I woke early and began to take a shower. I was washing my hair when I heard my mom screaming, "Daddy's dead! Daddy's dead!" I ran out out of the bathroom with a towel around me.

My mom screamed, "Get Pam!" (our next door neighbor.) I ran out of the house in my towel, with shampoo still in my hair. Pam opened her door as I cried, "We think my dad is dead!" She followed me back to the house. After that, it is pretty much a blur. I know the ambulance came, but I can't remember seeing it or re-calling what anyone said. I am sure I was in shock. I still don't want to remember anything more of that day. What happened next that day and the days following is still a blur in my mind.

Some time later, my dad was in the hospital and I remember feeding him water through a pink sponge as he lay on a bed with his legs all bandaged up. I remember him looking pale. And then I remember, distinctly, thinking:

This isn't my father. I guess he died and they felt bad that four kids wouldn't have a father, so they tried to give us this guy as a substitute. I don't know who this man is, but he certainly is not my dad.

The stranger never smiled; he just lay there looking so fragile and distant. Still puzzled and scared, I held the sponge up to his cracked lips, and he drank from it.

A strange memory comes to my mind. It must have been many months later. I was twelve years old and was sitting down in a therapist's office. She kept asking me insulting questions like "Do you know how to spell ocean backwards?" I could feel that she was stalling. I knew this had something to do with my dad, but I really didn't understand what there was to say. Robin and Katelyn knew the truth about what happened to my dad but Ryan and I were told a different story. I had been told that he went to the hospital because he was feeling sick. They gave him the wrong medicine, and he got dizzy and fell down the steps. That was all there was to it. It was just a mistake. He broke his legs, but he was going to be fine.

After about ten similar questions, my mom came into the room and joined us. She then quietly told me that my father had not fallen down the stairs, but had instead tried to kill himself by jumping out of a window. I didn't believe it. I felt my face burning with anger, and ran out of the room.

Later, I went to several therapists, but I couldn't imagine how on earth my talking to some forty-year-old woman would help my father walk and feel better. I guess I didn't cooperate, for—as far as I was concerned—the two situations could not be less related.

My mom was certain that we needed to talk about it to get the emotions out of us—like leeches for bad blood in the Middle Ages. We would be seated in the mini-van and, somehow, my mom would bring it up. I just hated talking about it! I hated thinking about it! And I especially hated how everyone kept harping on the idea that if we spent a certain quota of hours just talking about it, we'd feel better.

When my dad came home from the hospital, both his legs were broken, so he couldn't walk. The hospital bed was in the living room. I remember making him huge bowls of oatmeal—about seven or eight packets at a time—and carrying them in to him. And I remember the pills: at least a dozen orange bottles with lids of white all lined up on a shelf in the kitchen.

For a while after everything happened, the neighbors kept sending casseroles and making us dinner. We would dine well every night on buttered spaghetti or lasagna, but it didn't change anything. Our former life was gone and the worse was yet to come.

One day my parents called us all downstairs. They calmly told us that they were going to get divorced! It was a huge shock. I never thought that was a possibility with my family because we were all so close and I had never even seen my parents so much as argue. It couldn't be true! I wasn't ready for it! What more could happen to us!

I remember my dad crying on the side of his bed, with his eyes puffy and pink. I couldn't understand why he was leaving. And no one would explain. It seemed like a sort of double-edged sword. Everyone kept asking, "Do you want to talk about it?" And when I finally would ask a question, they quickly assured me, "You wouldn't understand, you're just a little kid."

I don't have any more to say. Things have changed again and life is more serene. We are back together. I'm just glad I have my dad. I have no idea where I would be without him. He was my basketball coach before and after, always believing in me and encouraging me in everything I did. He and my mom have always been my rock . . . and I have grown.

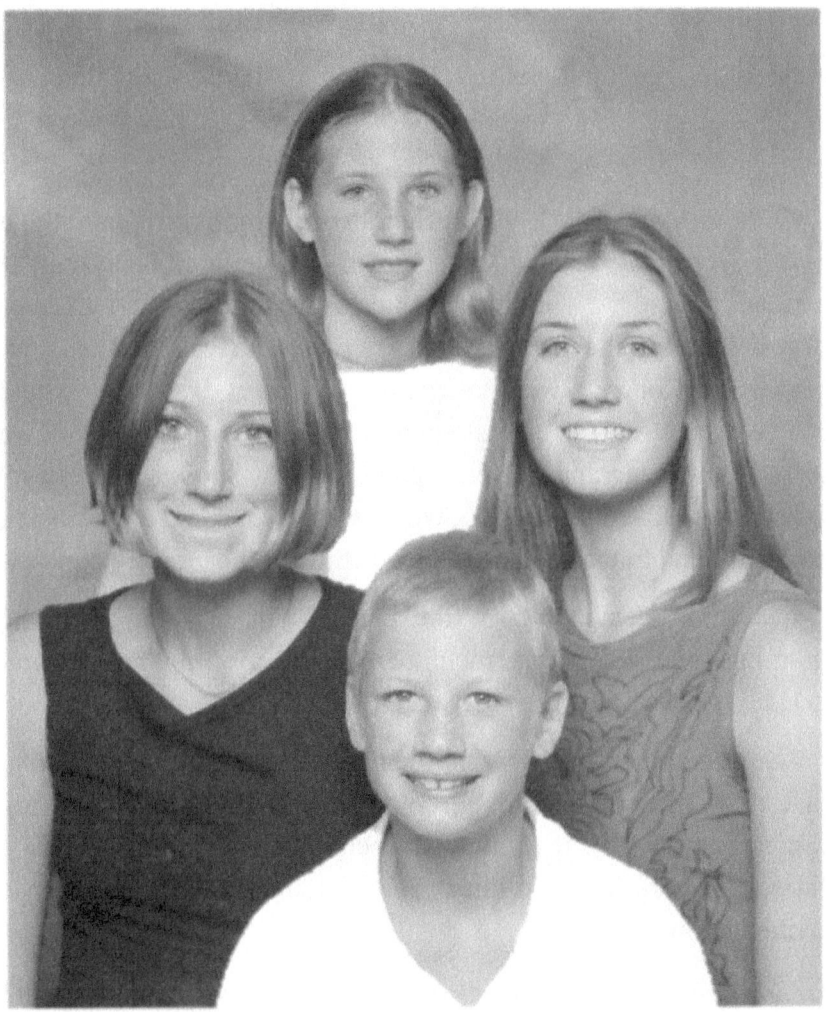

This is a photo taken at Walmart the week before the tragedy.

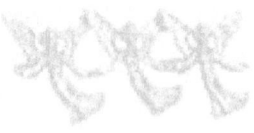

Ryan's Story

On March 20, 1999, I celebrated my ninth birthday with a birthday cake and presents; my whole family was there. I was just a normal little kid in the third grade. I liked to play baseball in the back yard with my friends Evan, Matt and my best friend Robert. I went to Richboro Elementary School, where my favorite class—like most young boys'—was gym. In gym, we tossed bean bags and played a game called "Shoot the Turkey." Of course, I loved recess, too, where we played kickball, baseball, and two-hand touch football, and we climbed the monkey bars.

Nothing seemed out of the ordinary in my life until one morning, the following month, I heard my mother scream, "Daddy's dead!" and then "Ryan, call 911!"

Scared and crying, I dialed the number. I ran for an angel pin, that lay in piles on the dining room table, and tried to get into my dad's room to give it to him. My neighbor hugged me and then shooed me back downstairs. Soon afterwards, an ambulance arrived in our driveway.

My mother had called her best friend a few minutes earlier, in a panic. She took me over to her house until my grandparents came and they took me to school.

I stayed at school all of that day and then my grandfather picked me up and took me to his house in Chalfont. Things happened that night at about 7:30 p.m., but I was not aware of anything wrong until the next day when my mother told me that my father had to stay in the hospital because he "fell down a flight of stairs and crushed both of his legs." She calmed me down and did not say anything to frighten me. Still, I was frightened later on, when I went to the hospital to visit him and saw him lying on the bed looking like a mummy. I dashed out of the room!

The days after that are a blur to me. The next thing I remember is that we had a refrigerator full of food supplied by the neighbors. We had so much that my mother finally had to ask them kindly to stop. My best friend Robert and his dad took me to lots of baseball games.

After my dad came home, he eventually was able to use a wheel chair. I remember playing catch with him. It was just like our normal times except that now I would have to chase the balls. My dad couldn't stand up or walk yet. He was brought to all my baseball games by our neighbor and good friend who would also pick up my dad every day and take him for therapy in Langhorne.

As far as I was concerned, things seemed to be going okay around the house. But then, for some reason unknown to me, my dad went to live with his sister. That is when turmoil entered my young life.

Several months later, my dad moved to his father's apartment in Lawndale. I still saw my dad, but transportation made it difficult for me to see him as much as we would like. He lived about 45 minutes away from us. By this time, he had a job as front end man-ager at a sporting goods store, and he seemed to be getting along great—although he was not at home with us. I missed being a part of my dad's life. I would call often, but the bottom line is that April 30, 1999, drastically changed my life.

Mom - Mom's Story

On April 30,1999, I received the most shocking news in my entire seventy-two years of life. The phone rang as we were finishing dinner. I guess it was about 7:30 p.m. Our two grand-children, Kristen and Ryan, had finished eating and were upstairs playing a game. The Caller ID told us it was Warminster Hospital. I picked up the phone and heard Trisha's voice. There was nothing unusual about that either—until she screamed out the words,

"JOHN JUST JUMPED OUT THE WINDOW!"

I knew she had taken him to the Emergency Room, as she had called that morning in a panic because she had found John unconscious in bed. Just a few minutes before the panic stricken phone call, she called very calmly and asked us to bring John a pair of socks to the hospital. She also asked us to drop the two younger children off. It had been a rough morning and she wanted the kids to all be home with her—safe and sound in their own beds. Now, there would be no "dropping Kristen and Ryan" off. My husband dashed to his car and flew to the hospital. I was glued to the spot. I couldn't leave with him. The kids, who were 9 and 12 years old, came down and asked where Granddad was.

I said, "He had to go somewhere, but the good news is that your mother called and said you can stay all night." This made them happy, and they went back to their play.

I was in a frenzy. *How could John do this? Was he already dead? Would he die? How badly was he injured? How was Trisha doing?*

There was no answer to those questions. I had to wait until Bob called me.

Slowly, I got back to doing routine tasks. I cleared the table and did the dishes. I called the kids down, and we played a game on the kitchen table. All the while, I attempted to stay calm. I did not want to frighten them. After a while, we had a milk-shake and some cookies, and I put them to bed.

As soon as I had a chance, I called my daughter Joann. Bob had called our other daughter, Janice, on his cell phone. She and Jim had already driven to the hospital. Joann said she would come and take me. I had to find someone to stay with Kristen and Ryan, who were now asleep. When I called my friend Millie, she immediately agreed to come over and stay until I came home. I hopped into Joann's car, and we drove to the hospital—as quickly as the law would allow. By this time, it was after 11 o'clock.

When we got there, all our family, including John's sister and her husband sat quietly waiting. John was in surgery. There wasn't much conversation. Everyone was silently praying, aware that John—in jumping three stories to the sidewalk—had crushed his legs almost beyond repair, and had sustained other injuries to his head and body.

After hours of waiting, the surgeon, clad in green, strode into the room. All eyes and ears were on him. He said he had worked on John's legs, and that he believed that John would be able to walk again. He did not mention any other injuries.

He was alive! That seemed, at the moment, to be all that mattered. No one realized all the agony that he would have to go through in the weeks and months ahead, or how it would affect all of his family.

Of course, there had been signs that led up to this moment. Trisha had called us more than once, when she had to take John to the hospital. Although we were concerned, we never dreamed how serious it all was, or that it would culminate in his serious desire to die.

Some things had seemed strange to us in the weeks prior to all this. When Trisha, John, and the family would drop in early on a school night to visit, John would nod off as he sat on the couch.

The four children seemed tired, too. Silently, we wondered, since they would stay till after 10:00, why they all weren't home in bed. We didn't know what was going on, as Trisha never spoke much about the problems taking place at home. She didn't mention much about John's concern about losing this job. Or, if she did, we did not take it seriously. We did notice John doing some things that didn't seem right. Once he told me he had decided to start cooking and needed some of my recipes; then, the next time he came, he didn't even mention it.

In the days after the accident, Bob and I often visited John, but we didn't talk to him about what he had done. We didn't want to upset him. Trisha was there every day, and we would often be at their house caring for the kids. Finally, John came home, unable to walk; he was confined to the hospital bed in the living room.

We were not privy to much that went on in the following days, but I know that the load was too much for Trisha. She seemed to have a need to get out of the house. Often when we called, she was not there and no one knew where she was. The whole situation was getting to her and, although we didn't realize it, she was going to support groups or therapy for herself.

98

This was the beginning of the "fall of the house of Gallagher." The words "John jumped out the window" echoed for years—as the family slowly began to fall apart.

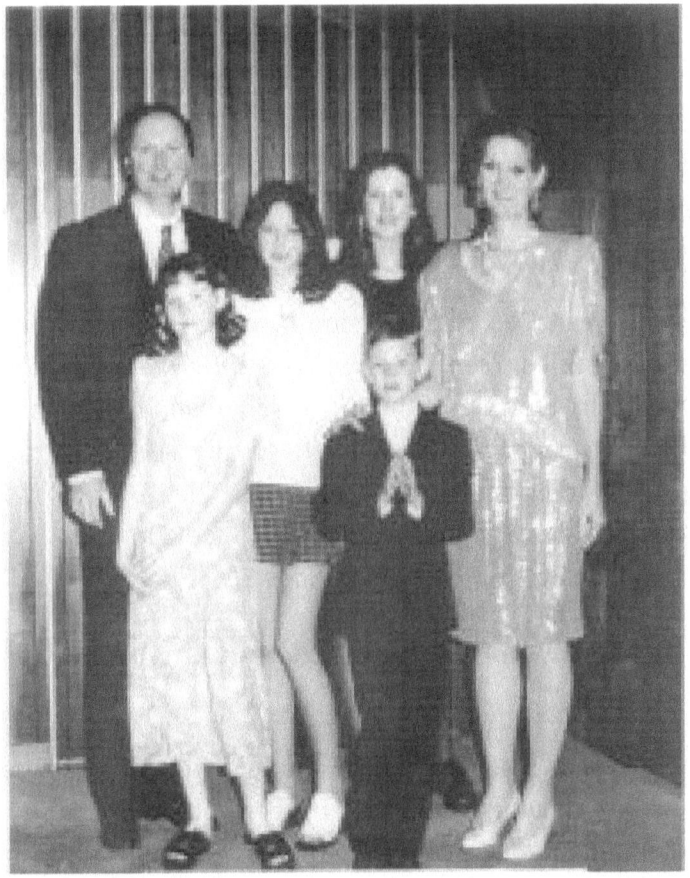

Are There Any Questions?

Does Oprah know that the family she touted as HAPPY and featured on her show twice shattered a few years later?

Several years before depression ravaged our family, my wife wrote a book titled *Raising Happy Kids on a Reasonable Budget.* The Oprah film crew came out to our suburban Philadelphia home and filmed a segment which aired on the show. Then Oprah arranged for Trisha and Katelyn to fly to Chicago to be guests on the show. The show reran a year later. We sent Oprah an email but we have not heard from the Oprah Show.

Why did your family tell everybody that you had been in a car accident?

There is such a stigma attached to the word *suicide*. We were beyond shock that this could have happened to us. I was so logical and just a regular type of dad. All of this seemed so unbelievable. We were very active in our community and I guess we just didn't want anybody to judge our family and talk about us. What we have learned through all of this is to never judge anyone. You never know what a person or a family is going through, unless you "have walked in their shoes."

Why didn't you even tell your father the truth?

My father was at the beginning stages of Alzheimer's. I was so embarrassed about the possibility of losing my job and I didn't want my father or father-in-law to know about the corporate downsizing. I guess my identity was tied to being a good provider and protector, the same values I learned from them. Losing the job made me feel like a failure.

What has been the impact of your secrecy on your four children?

It was hard because we did not tell extended family, friends, neighbors and church members what had really happened. We told them to say I was in an accident. This led to them isolating from their friends because they were afraid they would say the wrong thing. It also taught them that depression was shameful.

What were the effects of living with a dad who had depression and a mom who was trying to pick up the pieces of the old life?

To the children, it was confusing. Their dad didn't want to talk about anything and their mom wanted to talk about it a lot. We separated, and three of the kids moved to a new town with Trisha. Robin moved in with Mom-Mom. I lived about 45 minutes away from them for about a year. Then, I moved to an apartment a few minutes from their house. New schools, new friends, and a new lifestyle but we all adjusted and thrived. I am so very proud of all of them.

After a five year marital separation, what reunited you and your wife?

We had a crisis with one of our children.

Why did your family decide to write a book titled *NO MORE SECRETS - A FAMILY SPEAKS ABOUT DEPRESSION, ANXIETY AND ATTEMPTED SUICIDE?*

On January 20, I read a feature story in the Philadelphia Inquirer about a young man who had jumped nine stories from an apartment building. "Out of the blue" that day, I said, "I am not going to let this happen to one more family. I am going to write a book. I said to Trish, "Can you call all of the kids to our house for dinner tonight? I want them each to write a chapter." Katelyn and Trisha were willing participants. They had been waiting for years to be able to share how all of this affected them. Robin said, "Dad, I don't remember anything. That was so long ago." She once remarked, "Dad, I spent so much time trying to forget about it, I don't want to try to remember." When she did write her chapter, she was very honest and open. Katelyn asked if she could do some of the photos for the book. She added, "Dad, I would take a picture of our house on Holly Hill Road and turn it upside down. And then, I would take a family photo from that year and turn it upside down. Because that is how my life has felt since then....like it's been upside down." Kristen didn't want to talk much about it. For Kristen, it brought up a lot of transitions that still cause her pain. Her story helped us to understand life through the eyes of a twelve year old. Ryan, who was nine years old, was protected from much of what was going on. When they did write their chapters, they told of their unique memories. Ryan asked his grandmother for help in writing his chapter because he couldn't recall his feelings. I guess my personal sharing was helpful for them to read. We have learned so much. They know now that I was not abandoning them or being "selfish" by attempting suicide. I honestly don't know if my children will read the book, but by simply talking about it, for the past year, we are no longer in the dark about how each of us felt. The book has been the start of healing for all of us.

How is your family now?

I currently work in a men's clothing store and the four kids (all young adults) are in college, all studying psychology. Trisha and I founded the *Speaking About Depression Initiative*. Our mission is to carry our message about *Real Men, Real Depression* to organizations, church groups, retreats, and corporate meetings—locally, nationally and worldwide.

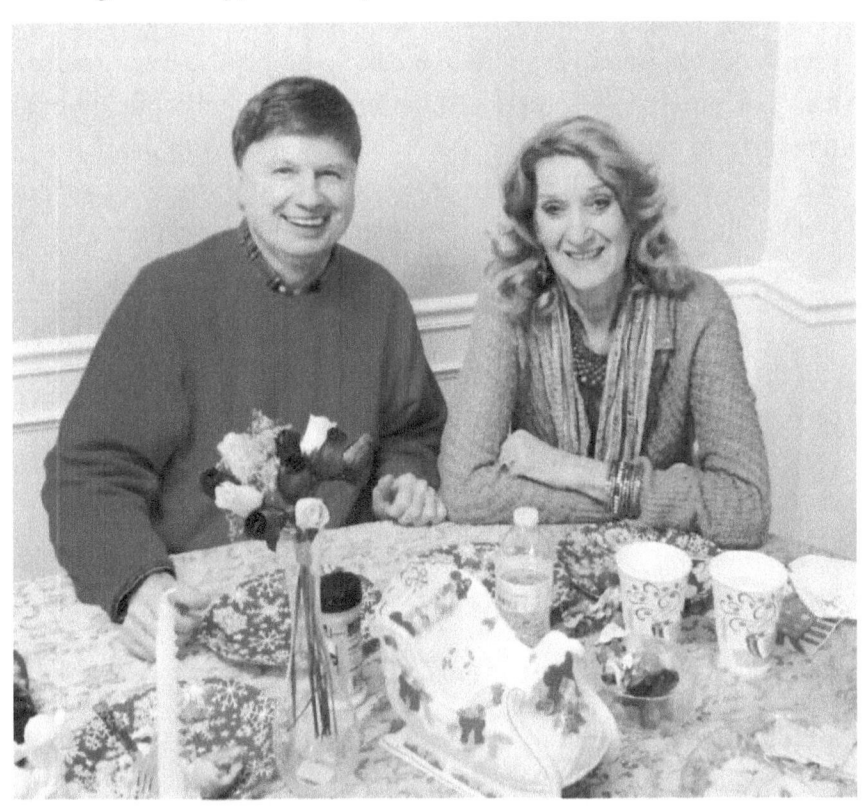

Frequently Asked Questions about Depression

What Is Depression?

Everyone occasionally feels blue or sad, but these feelings are usually fleeting and pass within a couple of days. When a person has a depressive disorder, it interferes with daily life, normal functioning, and causes pain for both the person with the disorder and those who care about him or her. Depression is a common but serious illness, and most who experience it need treatment to get better.

Many people with a depressive illness never seek treatment. But the vast majority, even those with the most severe depression, can get better with treatment. Intensive research into the illness has resulted in the development of medications, psychotherapies, and other methods to treat people with this disabling disorder.

Depression is a common but serious illness. Most who experience depression need treatment to get better.

What are the different forms of depression?

There are several forms of depressive disorders. The most common are major depressive disorder and dysthymic disorder.

Major depressive disorder, also called major depression, is characterized by a combination of symptoms that interfere with a person's ability to work, sleep, study, eat, and enjoy oncepleasurable activities. Major depression is disabling and prevents a person from functioning normally. An episode of major depression may occur only once in a person's lifetime, but more often, it recurs throughout a person's life.

Dysthymic disorder, also called dysthymia, is characterized by longterm (two years or longer) but less severe symptoms that may not disable a person but can prevent one from functioning normally or feeling well. People with dysthymia may also experience one or more episodes of major depression during their lifetimes.

Some forms of depressive disorder exhibit slightly different characteristics than those described above, or they may develop under unique circumstances. However, not all scientists agree on how to characterize and define these forms of depression.

They include:

Psychotic depression, which occurs when a severe depressive illness is accompanied by some form of psychosis, such as a break with reality, hallucinations, and delusions.

Postpartum depression, which is diagnosed if a new mother develops a major depressive episode within one month after delivery. It is estimated that 10 to 15 percent of women experience postpartum depression after giving birth.

Seasonal affective disorder (SAD), which is characterized by the onset of a depressive illness during the winter months, when there is less natural sunlight. The depression generally lifts during spring and summer. SAD may be effectively treated with light therapy, but nearly half of those with SAD do not respond to light therapy alone. Antidepressant medication and psychotherapy can reduce SAD symptoms, either alone or in combination with light therapy.

Bipolar disorder, also called manic-depressive illness, is not as common as major depression or dysthymia. Bipolar disorder is characterized by cycling mood changes—from extreme highs (e.g., mania) to extreme lows (e.g., depression). More information about bipolar disorder is available at http://www.nimh.nih.gov/health information/bipolarmenu.cfm.

What are the symptoms of depression?

People with depressive illnesses do not all experience the same symptoms. The severity, frequency and duration of symptoms will vary depending on the individual and his or her particular illness.

Persistent sad, anxious or "empty" feelings

Feelings of hopelessness and/or pessimism

Feelings of guilt, worthlessness and/or helplessness

Irritability, restlessness

Loss of interest in activities or hobbies once pleasurable, including sex

Fatigue and decreased energy

Difficulty concentrating, remembering details and making decisions

Insomnia, early-morning wakefulness, or excessive sleeping

Overeating, or appetite loss

Thoughts of suicide, suicide attempts

Persistent aches or pains, headaches, cramps or digestive problems that do not ease even with treatment

What illnesses often co-exist with depression?

Depression often co-exists with other illnesses. Such illnesses may precede the depression, cause it, and/or be a consequence of it. It is likely that the mechanics behind the intersection of depression and other illnesses differ for every person and situation. Regardless, these other co-occurring illnesses need to be diagnosed and treated.

Anxiety disorders, such as post-traumatic stress disorder (PTSD), obsessive-compulsive disorder, panic disorder, so-cial phobia and generalized anxiety disorder, often accompany depression. People experiencing PTSD are especially prone to having co-occurring depression. PTSD is a debilitating condition that can result after a person experiences a terrifying event or ordeal, such as a violent assault, a natural disaster, an accident, terrorism or military combat. People with PTSD often relive the traumatic event in flashbacks, memories or nightmares. Other symptoms include irritability, anger outbursts, intense guilt, and avoidance of thinking or talking about the traumatic ordeal. In a National Institute of Mental Health (NIMH)-funded study, researchers found that more than 40 percent of people with PTSD also had depression at one-month and four-month intervals after the traumatic event.

Alcohol and other substance abuse or dependence may also co-occur with depression. In fact, research has indicated that the co-existence of mood disorders and substance abuse is pervasive among the U.S. population.

Depression also often co-exists with other serious medical illnesses such as heart disease, stroke, cancer, HIV Aids, diabetes, and Parkinson's disease. Studies have shown that people who have depression in addition to another serious medical illness tend to have more severe symptoms of both depression and the medical illness, more difficulty adapting to their medical condition, and more medical costs than those who do not have co-existing depression. Research has yielded increasing evidence that treating the depression can also help improve the outcome of treating the co-occurring illness.

What causes depression?

There is no single known cause of depression. Rather, it likely results from a combination of genetic, biochemical, environmental, and psychological factors.

Research indicates that depressive illnesses are disorders of the brain. Brain-imaging technologies, such as magnetic resonance imaging (MRI), have shown that the brains of people who have depression look different than those of people without depression. The parts of the brain responsible for regulating mood, thinking, sleep, appetite and behavior appear to function abnormally. In addition, important neurotransmitters—chemicals that brain cells use to communicate—appear to be out of balance. But these images do not reveal **why** the depression has occurred. Some types of depression tend to run in families, suggesting a genetic link. However, depression can occur in people without family histories of depression as well. Genetics research indicates that risk for depression results from the influence of multiple genes acting together with environmental or other factors. In addition, trauma, loss of a loved one, a difficult relationship, or any stressful situation may trigger a depressive episode. Subsequent depressive episodes may occur with or without an obvious trigger. *Research indicates that depressive illnesses are disorders of the brain.*

How do women experience depression?

Depression is more common among women than among men. Biological, life cycle, hormonal and psychosocial factors unique to women may be linked to women's higher depression rate. Researchers have shown that hormones directly affect brain chemistry that controls emotions and mood. For example, women are particularly vulnerable to depression after giving birth, when hormonal and physical changes, along with the new responsibility of caring for a newborn, can be overwhelming. Many new mothers experience a brief episode of the "baby blues," but some will develop postpartum depression, a much more serious condition that requires active treatment and emotional support for the new mother. Some studies suggest that women who experience post-partum depression often have had prior depressive episodes.

Some women may also be susceptible to a severe form of pre-menstrual syndrome (PMS), sometimes called premenstrual dysphoric disorder (PMDD), a condition resulting from the hormonal changes that typically occur around ovulation and before menstruation begins. During the transition into menopause, some women experience an increased risk for depression. Scientists are exploring how the cyclical rise and fall of estrogen and other hormones may affect the brain chemistry that is associated with depressive illness.

Finally, many women face the additional stresses of work and home responsibilities, caring for children and aging parents, abuse, poverty, and relationship strains. It remains unclear why some women faced with enormous challenges develop depression, while others with similar challenges do not.

How do men experience depression?

Men often experience depression differently than women and may have different ways of coping with the symptoms. Men are more likely to acknowledge having fatigue, irritability, loss of in-terest in once-pleasurable activities, and sleep disturbances, whereas women are more likely to admit to feelings of sadness, worthlessness and/or excessive guilt.

Men are more likely than women to turn to alcohol or drugs when they are depressed, or become frustrated, discouraged, irritable, angry and sometimes abusive. Some men throw themselves into their work to avoid talking about their depression with family or friends, or engage in reckless, risky behavior. And even though more women attempt suicide, many more men die by suicide in the United States.

How do older adults experience depression?

Depression is not a normal part of aging, and studies show that most seniors feel satisfied with their lives, despite increased physical ailments. However, when older adults do have depression, it may be overlooked because seniors may show different, less obvious symptoms, and may be less inclined to experience or acknowledge feelings of sadness or grief. In addition, older adults may have more medical conditions such as heart disease, stroke or cancer, which may cause depressive symptoms, or they may be taking medications with side effects that contribute to depression. Some older adults may experience what some doctors call vascular depression, also called arteriosclerotic depression or subcortical ischemic depression. Vascular depression may result when blood vessels become less flexible and harden over time, becoming constricted. Such hardening of vessels prevents normal blood flow to the body's organs, including the brain. Those with vascular depression may have, or be at risk for, a co-existing cardiovascular illness or stroke. Although many people assume that the highest rates of suicide are among the young, older white males age 85 and older actually have the highest suicide rate. Many have a depressive illness that their doctors may not detect, despite the fact that these suicide victims often visit their doctors within one month of their deaths. The majority of older adults with depression improve when they receive treatment with an antidepressant, psychotherapy, or a combination of both. Research has shown that medication alone and combination treatment are both effective in reducing the rate of depressive recurrences in older adults.

Psychotherapy alone also can be effective in prolonging periods free of depression, especially for older adults with minor depression, and it is particularly useful for those who are unable or un-willing to take antidepressant medication. *Depression is not a normal part of aging.*

How do children and adolescents experience depression?

Scientists and doctors have begun to take seriously the risk of depression in children. Research has shown that childhood depression often persists, recurs and continues into adulthood, especially if it goes untreated. The presence of childhood depression also tends to be a predictor of more severe illnesses in adulthood. A child with depression may pretend to be sick, refuse to go to school, cling to a parent, or worry that a parent may die. Older children may sulk, get into trouble at school, be negative and irritable, and feel misunderstood. Because these signs may be viewed as normal mood swings typical of children as they move through developmental stages, it may be difficult to accurately diagnose a young person with depression.

Before puberty, boys and girls are equally likely to develop depressive disorders. By age 15, however, girls are twice as likely as boys to have experienced a major depressive episode. Depression in adolescence comes at a time of great personal change—when boys and girls are forming an identity distinct from their parents, grappling with gender issues and emerging sexuality, and making decisions for the first time in their lives. Depression in adolescence frequently co-occurs with other disorders such as anxiety, disruptive behavior, eating disorders or substance abuse. It can also lead to increased risk for suicide.

An NIMH-funded clinical trial of 439 adolescents with major depression found that a combination of medication and psychotherapy was the most effective treatment option. Other

NIMH-funded researchers are developing and testing ways to prevent suicide in children and adolescents, including early diagnosis and treatment, and a better understanding of suicidal thinking. *Childhood depression often persists, recurs, and continues into adulthood, especially if left untreated.*

How is depression detected and treated?

Depression, even the most severe cases, is a highly treatable disorder. As with many illnesses, the earlier that treatment can begin, the more effective it is and the greater the likelihood that recurrence can be prevented.

The first step to getting appropriate treatment is to visit a doctor. Certain medications, and some medical conditions such as viruses or a thyroid disorder, can cause the same symptoms as depression. A doctor can rule out these possibilities by conducting a physical examination, interview and lab tests. If the doctor can eliminate a medical condition as a cause, he or she should conduct a psychological evaluation or refer the patient to a mental health professional.

The doctor or mental health professional will conduct a complete diagnostic evaluation. He or she should discuss any family history of depression, and get a complete history of symptoms, e.g., when they started, how long they have lasted, their severity, and whether they have occurred before and if so, how they were treated. He or she should also ask if the patient is using alcohol or drugs, and whether the patient is thinking about death or suicide

How can I help a friend or relative who is depressed?

If you know someone who is depressed, it affects you too. The first and most important thing you can do to help a friend or relative who has depression is to help him or her get an appropriate diagnosis and treatment. You may need to make an appointment on behalf of your friend or relative and go with him or her to see the doctor. Encourage him or her to stay in treatment, or to seek different treatment if no improvement occurs after six to eight weeks.

Offer emotional support, understanding, patience and encouragement.

Engage your friend or relative in conversation, and listen carefully. Never disparage feelings your friend or relative expresses, but point out realities and offer hope.

Never ignore comments about suicide, and report them to your friend's or relative's therapist or doctor.

Invite your friend or relative out for walks, outings and other activities. Keep trying if he or she declines, but don't push him or her to take on too much too soon. Although diversions and company are needed, too many demands may increase feelings of failure.

Remind your friend or relative that with time and treatment, the depression will lift.

How can I help myself if I am depressed?

If you have depression, you may feel exhausted, helpless and hopeless. It may be extremely difficult to take any action to help yourself. But it is important to realize that these feelings are part of the depression and do not accurately reflect actual circumstances. As you begin to recognize your depression and begin treatment, negative thinking will fade.

Engage in mild activity or exercise. Go to a movie, a ballgame, or another event or activity that you once enjoyed. Participate in religious, social or other activities.

Set realistic goals for yourself.

Break up large tasks into small ones, set some priorities and do what you can as you can.

Try to spend time with other people and confide in a trusted friend or relative. Try not to isolate yourself, and let others help you.

Expect your mood to improve gradually, not immediately. Do not expect to suddenly "snap out of" your depression. Often during treatment for depression, sleep and appetite will begin to improve before your depressed mood lifts.

Postpone important decisions, such as getting married or divorced or changing jobs, until you feel better. Discuss decisions with others who know you well and have a more objective view of your situation.

Remember that positive thinking will replace negative thoughts as your depression responds to treatment.

Where can I go for help?

If you are unsure where to go for help, ask your family doctor. Others who can help are listed below.

- Mental health specialists, such as psychiatrists, psychologists, social workers, or mental health counselors

- Health maintenance organizations Community mental health centers

- Hospital psychiatry departments and outpatient clinics Mental health programs at universities or medical schools State hospital outpatient clinics

- Family services, social agencies or clergy Peer support groups

- Private clinics and facilities Employee assistance programs

- Local medical and/or psychiatric societies

You can also check the phone book under "mental health," "health," "social services," "hotlines," or "physicians" for phone numbers and addresses. An emergency room doctor also can provide temporary help and can tell you where and how to get further help.

What if I or someone I know is in crisis?

If you are thinking about harming yourself, or know someone who is, tell someone who can help immediately.

- Call your doctor.

- Call 911 or go to a hospital emergency room to get immediate help or ask a friend or family member to help you do these things.

- Call the toll-free, 24-hour hotline of the National Suicide Prevention Lifeline at 1 800-273-TALK (1 800-273-8255).

- Make sure you or the suicidal person is not left alone.

Resources

This is by no means an exhaustive list but the following organizations, books, resources and web sites may be useful. Please do not use these resources as a substitute for medical and psychological care. They are simply an adjunct to your personal research and professional support.

Organizations

American Academy of Child and Adolescent Psychiatry 3615 Wisconsin Ave., N.W.
Washington, D.C. 20016 (202) 966-7300
Internet: *http://www.aacap.org*

American Mental Health Counseling Association 801 N. Fairfax St., Suite 304
Alexandria, VA 22314 (800) 326-2642
Internet: *http://www.amhca.org*

American Psychiatric Association Public Affairs Office, Suite 501 1400 K St., N.W.
Washington, D.C. 20005 (202) 682-6220
Internet: *http://www.psych.org*

American Psychological Association 750 First St., N.E.
Washington, D.C. 20002 (202) 336-5800
Internet: *http://helping.apa.org*

Anxiety Disorders Association of America 11900 Parklawn Dr., Suite 100
Rockville, MD 20852-2624 (301) 231-9350
Internet: *http://www.adaa.org/*

Association for Advancement of Behavior Therapy 305 Seventh Ave., 16th Floor
New York, NY 10001 (212) 647-1890
Freedom From Fear 308 Seaview Ave.
Staten Island, NY 10305 (718) 351-1717
Internet: *http://www.freedomfromfear.org*

National Institute of Mental Health Public Inquiries, Rm. 8184, MSC 9663 6001 Executive Blvd.
Bethesda, MD 20892
National Alliance for the Mentally Ill 200 N. Glebe Rd., Suite 1015 Arlington, VA 22201
(800) 950-NAMI
Internet: *http://www.nami.org*

NAMI is the National Alliance on Mental Illness, the nation's largest grassroots organization for people with mental illness and their families. Founded in 1979, NAMI has affiliates in every state and in more than 1,100 local communities across the country. NAMI recognizes that the key concepts of recovery, resiliency and support are essential to improving the wellness and quality of life of all persons affected by mental illness. Mental illnesses should not be an obstacle to a full and meaningful life for persons who live with them. NAMI advocates at all levels to ensure that all persons affected by mental illness receive the services that they need and deserve, in a timely fashion. For help in finding self-help groups, NAMI can provide phone numbers of state and regional chapters and affiliates in your area.

National Anxiety Foundation 3135 Custer Dr.
Lexington, KY 40517-4001
National Council on Alcoholism and Drug Dependence (NCADD)
12 West 21st Street New York, NY 10010 (800) NCA-CALL
Internet address: *http://www.ncadd.org*
National Institute on Alcohol Abuse and Alcoholism Scientific

Communications Branch
6000 Executive Boulevard, Suite 409 Bethesda, MD 20892-7003
(301) 443-3860
Internet address: *http://www.niaaa.nih.gov*

National Association of Social Workers Clinical Registrar Office
750 First St., N.E., Suite 700
Washington, D.C. 20002-4241 (800) 638-8799
Internet: *http://www.naswdc.org*

Depression and Bipolar Support Alliance
730 N. Franklin, Suite 501
Chicago, IL 60610 (800) 826-3632
Internet Address: *www.dbsa.org*

The mission of the Depression and Bipolar Support Alliance (DBSA) is to provide hope, help, and support to improve the lives of people living with depression or bipolar disorder. DBSA pursues and accomplishes this mission through peerbased, recovery-oriented, empowering services and resources *when* people want them, *where* they want them, and *how* they want them.

Mental Health America (formerly National Mental Health Association)
1021 Prince St.
Alexandria, VA 22314-2971
(703) 684-7722 or (800) 969-NMHA
Internet: www.mentalhealthamerica.com

Obsessive Compulsive Foundation 9 Depot St.
Milford, CT 06460 (203) 878-5669
Internet: *http://pages.prodigy.com/alwillen/ocf.html*

Self-Help Groups

ABIL, Inc. (Agoraphobics Building Independent Lives)
3805 Cutshaw Ave.
Suite 415
Richmond, VA 23230 (804) 353-3964
E-mail: *ABIL1996@aol.com*

A.I.M. (Agoraphobics in Motion) 1719 Crooks St.
Royal Oak, MI 48067-1306 (248) 547-0400
E-mail:anny@ameritech.net

American Self-Help Clearinghouse Northwest Covenant Medical Center 25 Pocono Rd.
Denville, NJ 07834 (800) 367-6724 (in NJ)
(201) 625-9565 (outside NJ)
Internet: *http://www.cmhc.com/selfhelp/*

Al-Anon Family Group Headquarters 1600 Corporate Landing Parkway Virginia Beach, VA 23454-5617
Internet address: *http://www.al-anon.alateen.org*

Locations of Al-Anon or Alateen meetings worldwide can be obtained by calling the toll-free numbers Monday through Friday, 8 a.m.-6 p.m. (e.s.t.):
U. S.: (800) 344-2666 Canada: (800) 443-4525

Free informational materials can be obtained by calling the toll-free numbers (operating 7 days a week, 24 hours per day):

U. S.: (800) 356-9996 Canada: (800) 714-7498
Alcoholics Anonymous (AA) World Services 475 Riverside Drive, 11th Floor
New York, NY 10115 (212) 870-3400
Internet address: *http://www.alcoholics-anonymous.org*

Makes referrals to local AA groups and provides informational materials on the AA program.
National Mental Health Self-Help Consumers Clearinghouse 1211 Chestnut St.
Suite 1000 Philadelphia, PA
(800) 553-4539 or (215) 735-1810
Internet: *http://www.libertynet.org/~mha/cl_house.html*

Phobics Anonymous P.O. Box 1180
Palm Springs, CA 92263 (619) 322-COPE

Recovery, Inc.
802 N. Dearborn St.
Chicago, IL 60610 (312) 337-5661

This information is available courtesy of the National Institute for Mental Health. For more information go to *http://www.nimh.nih.gov/practitioners/patinfo.cfm*

Information from NIMH is available in multiple formats. You can browse online, download documents in PDF, and order paper brochures through the mail. If you would like to have NIMH publications, you can order them online at *www.nimh.nih.gov*. If you do not have Internet access and wish to have information that supplements this publication, please contact the NIMH Information Center at the numbers listed below.

Please check the *NIMH Web site* for the most up-to-date information on this topic.

National Institute of Mental Health
Science Writing, Press & Dissemination Branch
6001 Executive Boulevard
Room 8184, MSC 9663 Bethesda, MD 20892-9663
Phone: 301-443-4513 or 1-866-615-NIMH (6464)

120

Toll-free TTY: 301-443-8431
TTY: 866-415-8051
FAX: 301-443-4279 E-mail: *nimhinfo@nih.gov*
Web site: *http://www.nimh.nih.gov*

Need some help in a hurry?

These are some websites that provide excellent information.
www.dbsalliance.org
www.mayoclinic.com
www.johnshopkinshealthalerts.com
www.postpartum.net
www.depression-primarycare.org
www.nmha.org
www.nami.org
www.fda.org
www.healthyminds.org
www.nimh.gov
www.nih.gov

Additional Sources of Support

www.afsp.org American Friends for Suicide Prevention
www.nmha.org Mental Health America, the country's oldest and largest non-profit organization addressing all aspects of mental health. A primary goal of Mental Health America is to educate the general public about the realities of mental health and mental illness related to the following issues:

- Anxiety Disorders
- Children's Health
- Depression
- Bipolar Disorder
- Eating Disorders
- Older Adults
- Other Illnesses
- Recovery
- Schizophrenia
- Suicide

www.mhlg.org Mental Health Liaison Group, a coalition of national organizations representing consumers, families, members, advocates, professionals and providers.

www.nlbha.org National Latino Behavioral Health Association, provides national leadership for the advancement of Latino behavioral health services.

www.suicidology.org American Association of Suicidology, The American Association of Suicidology (AAS) is a not-for-profit membership organization founded in 1968. AAS's mission is to understand and prevent suicide by: advancing Suicidology as a science and disseminating scholarly work in Suicidology, developing and implementing strategies to reduce the incidence and prevalence of suicidal behaviors, disseminating accurate public information about suicidal behaviors, fostering the highest possible quality of suicide prevention, intervention, and postvention to the public and promoting research, education, and training in Suicidology.

www.lifesaverstraining.org Lifesavers Training Corporation, a peer support, suicide and crisis-prevention program.

www.activeminds.org Active Minds on Campus, mental health awareness and advocacy on college campuses. Active Minds works to utilize the student voice to change the conversation about mental health on college campuses. By developing and supporting chapters of a studentrun mental health awareness, education, and advocacy group on campuses, the organization works to increase students' awareness of mental health issues, provide information and resources regarding mental health and mental illness, encourage students to seek help as soon as it is needed, and serve as liaison between students and the mental health community.

www.bazelon.org Bazelon Center for Mental Health Law, information on mental health resources and explanation of rights when seeking treatment.

www.mhreform.org The Campaign for Mental Health Reform, collaborative effort of 18 national mental health organizations to ensure that federal mental health policy is aligned with the fields collective vision.

www.familyaware.org Families for Depression Awareness, a non-profit organization that helps people understand mental health disorders and share issues. Families that work together are best able to cope with depressive disorders. Families for Depression Awareness helps people in caregiver roles and people with depressive disorders understand the conditions, reduce stigma, and share issues.

www.thelink.org The Link Counseling Center, a leading resource for suicide prevention and aftercare. Dedicated to reaching out to those whose lives have been impacted by suicide and connecting them to resources. Order excellent books at *www.boltonpress.com*

Recommended reading: My Son....My Son—A Guide to Healing After Death, Loss or Suicide by Iris Bolton.

www.suicidereferencelibrary.com   The   Suicide Reference Library

QPR Institute—a training organization that provides suicide prevention educational materials and programs to professionals and the general public.

www.samaritansnyc.org Samaritans USA, coalition whose principal purpose is to befriend people who are depressed, in crisis, or suicidal.

www.stopasuicide.org Stop A Suicide Today, developed by Harvard psychiatrist, Douglas Jacobs, MD.

www.save.org Suicide Awareness/Voices of Education, raises awareness and educates the public that suicide should no longer be a hidden or tabu topic.

www.sprc.org Suicide Prevention Resource Center, supports suicide prevention with the best of science, skills and practices.

www.suicidegrief.com   Suicide Grief Discussion Board

www.livingworks.net Living Works Education, suicide prevention and training intervention programs.

www.training.sprc.org National Center for Suicide Prevention Training, provides educational resources to help other coalitions develop effective suicide prevention programs and policies.

www.nopcas.org National Organization for People of Color Against Suicide, develops ideas that instill hope, improve health and save lives in communities of color.

www.preventingsuicide.com Preventing Suicide Network, a resource center aimed at providing authoritative and problem—specific information about suicide prevention.

www.jasonfoundation.com The Jason Foundation, Inc. (JFI) is a nationally recognized provider of educational curriculums and training programs for students, educators/youth workers and parents. JFI's programs build an awareness of the national health problem of youth suicide, educate participants in recognizing the "warning signs or signs of concern," provide information on identifying atrisk behavior and elevated risk groups, and direct participants to local resources to deal with possible suicidal ideation. JFI's student curriculums are presented in the "third-person" perspective—how to help a friend. The Jason Foundation, Inc. is a non-profit 501c3.

www.rebeccacutlerfoundation.org The Rebecca Lynn Cutler Legacy of Life Foundation was established in 2004 by Rebecca's

family in partnership with the Depression and Bipolar Support Alliance (DBSA). The Foundation is part of DBSA.

Rebecca's Dream is a foundation established by a loving family in honor of Rebecca Lynn Cutler, a vibrant, talented and successful young Chicago woman who lost her life to bipolar disorder. The foundation's mission is to foster awareness and compassionate understanding of depression and bipolar disorder as real diseases that affect real people like Rebecca and her family. Her family and DBSA are dedicated to keeping Rebecca's legacy alive by helping those who live with mood disorders—and their loved ones—know that there is hope.

No Kidding, Me Too! is an organization whose purpose is to remove the stigma attached to brain disease through education and the breaking down of societal barriers. Their goal is to empower those with brain disease to admit their illness, seek treatment, and become even greater members of society. They want a normal conversation in America to be:

"I have bipolar disorder/schizophrenia/insert disease" "No Kidding, Me Too!"

Joe Pantoliano (actor, Sopranos)
No Kidding, Me Too
210 West Hamilton Ave. Suite 229
State College, PA 16801 917-400-1036
Email: *Info@NoKiddingMeToo.org*
www.karlasmithfoundation.org

The Karla Smith Foundation, provides hope for a balanced life to family and friends of anyone with a mental illness or who lost a loved one to suicide. The Karla Smith Foundation, founded by Tom, her father, Fran, her mother, and Kevin, her twin brother, is an avenue to share family experiences which similarly impact thousands of others.

Recommended book: *A Balanced Life: 9 Strategies for Coping With the Mental Health Problem of a Loved One* by Thomas J. Smith. 1-800-KSF-HOPE. *www.jedfoundation.org* The Jed Foundation, was founded in 2000 by Donna and Phil Satow after they lost their son Jed to suicide.

While trying to learn more about suicide and make sense of their unthinkable loss, the Satows discovered an urgent and unmet need for programming and resources that helped colleges, students and parents recognize and address the signs of emotional distress and suicide.. *www.yellowribbon.org* Yellow Ribbon Suicide Prevention Campaign was founded in 1994 by Dale and Dar Emme, the parents of a bright, funny, loving teen, Mike Emme, who took his life when he did not know the words to say, or how to let someone know he was in trouble and needed help. Please see their website for the story of the Legacy of the Yellow Mustang, a poignant story of the beginning of their campaign.

The Link's National Resource Center for Suicide Prevention and Aftercare
348 Mt. Vernon Highway, NE
Atlanta, GA 30328
Website: *www.thelink.org*

The National Resource Center for Suicide Prevention and Aftercare is dedicated to reaching out to those affected by suicide and connecting them to resources. Suicide Prevention: through speeches and workshops concerning depression, warning signs of suicide, and how to respond and get help; resource materials including a Prevention Packet of Information; telephone counseling for individuals, family, and friends seeking support and guidance; information referrals concerning other resources and organizations; and suicide curriculum for high school students. Suicide Aftercare: referrals for support groups for survivors of suicide (SOS); telephone counseling for survivors and caregivers; SOS Support Team Training; resource materials including a Survivors of Suicide Packet of Information and The Journey, a survivor newsletter; and, information referrals concerning other resources and organizations.

National Suicide Prevention Lifeline 1-800-273-TALK (8255), provides immediate assistance to anyone seeking mental health services. Free and confidential. Call for yourself or someone you care about.

The Nicest Thing Somebody Ever Said or Did For Me

We want to encourage people to reach out and help someone struggling. We posed this question on the Internet, "What was the nicest thing someone ever said or did for you?" We hope that the readers of this book see that sometimes it is the little things that brighten a person's day... a kind word or deed, or just a simple breath of encouragement. We feel better ourselves when we do something nice for another. Perhaps, some of these heartwarming ideas will inspire you to help someone. Whether you are the one suffering with emotional pain, or the person caring for someone who has an illness, a little kindness can go a long way.

THE NICEST THING SAID TO ME

When a lady in church said, "God has something mighty planned for you." She gave me a laminated page of the 23rd Psalm. She didn't know me and maybe she said this to many people. It gave me a reason to hang on to hope. Even now, eight years later, I still reflect on those words for strength. It was at a time of great turmoil in my life and I desperately needed powerful words of encouragement.

"You can walk the road of life triumphantly, gloriously, as the radiant, victorious child of God, which you are."

I work in a business where, shall we say, a person's word is sometimes not entirely reliable. A colleague from another city said to me, "You know, Frank, if you'd tell me it's Christmas, I'd go hang up my stocking." Because I hold ethics and truthfulness as standards to aspire to, I took that as a real compliment.

"You changed my life! I will remember you until the day I die..." As a teacher, I sometimes lose heart due to loss of finances, as it is not the most lucrative profession. But when I see and hear what effect my work has on people, I am renewed with inspiration to keep on keepin' on all over again.

"You are a God wink. Thank you for being my friend."

"You're loved." The first time I heard it was from an elderly white woman (I'm African American) on a public bus. She was impressed by my kindness to her and the courtesies I extended (I gave her my seat). She said that she could look at me and tell somebody loved me. She said, "Yes, you're loved." And the second time was during dinner with a friend going through a tough time who said the exact same thing in the same context referencing the way I treated people and accepted them, flaws and all. The second time helped me recall the first time I heard it and gave me a point of observation with other people. I use those words to encourage people all of the time.

When I was 26, a friend of mine told me, "I would be happy if my daughter turned out to be like you one day." I was going through a difficult time in my life and it was very touching to hear. I can't imagine getting a higher compliment. He was in his 50's and his daughter was about 18 or 19.

I was tutoring an especially difficult set of twins. Their parents knew how difficult they were. Their negative self-image and lack of motivation were evident at home and at school. The parents decreased the hours they spent in their family businesses, and asked the kids about homework every night. I did all I could to motivate them. At the end of the year, the mother called to say that though their grades only went up slightly, "What you did for my children, as people, was worth every penny." I see tutoring as the vehicle through which I get to teach students about life. This was the highest compliment I'd ever received.

The nicest thing anyone ever said to me was: "Jillian, you make the room light up." Even now, my heart is singing from thinking about that person and what they said.

My father was in the final stages of brain cancer. We were not as close as we should be, and our lives were miles apart.

Following the brain surgery, I would go visit him as often as possible. His speech and memory had been affected, and what he said did not often make sense. One day after lunch with him, as we were saying our good-byes, we hugged. While hugging, I apologized for not being a better son. Through the pain and his inability to communicate clearly, he said, "Best son." I will never forget that.

I was talking to my husband's friend. She said that he speaks of me frequently, and he shares information about what is going on in our lives. What she said that took me completely by surprise was, "You are an inspiration." This shocked and pleased me because I am a fulltime working mother of three kids age 11, 7.5 and 6. Being an inspiration is not something I ever considered being capable of. When she said that we inspire her, it made me realize that the things I take for granted (a loving husband, three happy and healthy children, a 16 year marriage, etc.) have real value. And that somehow we had a positive impact on people around us.

My spiritual father would often tell me: "If God has picked you for promotion, he has first picked you for trial." Those words have brought comfort to me during the rough spots in my life. During a difficult time of my life, a wise pastor told me, "God is taking you to a place that you cannot see."

I had a moment one morning, where the crossing guard at my daughter's kindergarten said to me, "You are always smiling and happy." I responded "What's the alternative?" I never realized it was something others noticed. I enjoyed hearing it from a man that most people barely even recognized, but he and I would say a friendly "good morning" each day. It really made my day. I completely agree, little things said go a long way. I try, from my end, to say positive things to complete strangers, never knowing what impact it will have on them.

How I Fill My Love Tank When I Feel Depressed or Anxious

Just like a car needs a tank of fuel to keep it running efficiently, people need good things in their life to keep their spirit running optimally. They need their "love tank" filled! When I was recently feeling a little blue, my daughter said, "Mom, are you keeping your love tank filled?" It was a reminder to do some decorating, entertaining, and writing—the things that bring me contentment and joy. I asked people on the Internet to email as to how they keep their love tank filled. The following tips are expressed in their own unique ways:

HOW I FILL MY LOVE TANK

Take a nourishing bath with candles, rose petals, and bath salts. Prepare a healthy yummy treat and enjoy with a fun drink. Take a walk in my favorite place.

Go for a walk to look at nature. Buy myself a small treat or gift.

Take some time and read Psalm 23, line by line, and listen to the words. It's a Psalm of God's grace and mercy. When I'm going through something tough, I live in the book of Psalms.

Get some exercise. Go for a walk. Get on the treadmill. Do some yoga.

Take a deep breath and remind yourself that everything is going to be okay and that this too shall pass.

Engage in an affirmation and allow it to float gently in your mind and heart. Don't think about either accepting or rejecting it.

I don't let things bottle up inside of me. I speak the truth. I express my feelings and thoughts. When I am aggravated by an incident that takes me by surprise, I might say something out loud such as, "I am really angry because that other driver cut me off."

I am learning how to develop good communication skills so that I can deliver a skillful message explaining how someone's behavior is affecting me and how I feel about it. I use constructive comments. I use "I" messages.

I surrender to the Universe, to the flow of life. Breathe, relax and let be.

I ask myself, "What would I really love to do for myself today?" See what comes to mind. Is it possible to incorporate your wish somewhere in your day? Make time for whatever it is.

I take an evening walk.

I call a friend whom I haven't spoken to for awhile. I have a piece of cake.

I buy myself a little gift such as a CD of songs that I like.

I try to think of something that I really feel passionate about. I think about something I enjoy. It is important to cultivate these things in our daily lives—as a form of demonstrating love to our real self.

I use positive affirmations to focus on hopefulness, optimism and peace, rather than doubt, fear and anxiety. Affirmations are usually one-sentence statements such as the following: I am whole, complete, and perfect, just the way I am right now. I move forward with eager anticipation. I easily see the good in every situation.

I deserve happiness, and I claim it right now. Affirmations allow you to "switch channels" whenever your thoughts drift toward negative thinking.

I focus on empowering thoughts.

Humor therapy is a good way to "jump start" your sense of joy and happiness. Find reasons to laugh regularly.

Go to a funny movie, borrow one or rent one. Read the comics daily.

When I am depressed, I try the following: write or talk about what I am going through, whether it is on my blog, in a notebook, to a friend, to my counselor, to my pet parakeets, to God, or to myself. It just helps me emotionally to get it all out.

Sometimes when I feel like hurting myself or going down a negative road which causes me to spiral out of control, I will give my-self pep talks in my mind to prevent that from happening. I tell myself that I have the strength, and can get through this.

Have a virtual cup of tea with someone. Sip. Sip.

Looking at the sunset at Tahoe is awesome. Another sight that blew my mind was back in my days as a makeup artist. I was in Lancaster working on a film and the sunset was so fiery, it seemed to encompass the whole sky and, although I was dead tired from a long shoot, I had to stand there in the desert until the last wisps of color dissipated completely. There is something about looking up at the sky and realizing how small we are in this giant universe and, God knows what else out there. I'm going to dash out there now because I need a dose of humility.

I've talked to a hospice chaplain about this and he told me this was my tool to change my thoughts. I have seen the same advice in inspirational tapes and books such as *"Ask and It Shall Be Given."* It helped to bring me to that stage above depression. At my low-est points, I would get angry and that anger was directed at God. I screamed, "Why aren't you helping me?" It would make me get up out of bed and do something to bring me a notch above the depression. "I'll show you, God!" Twice when this happened,

I didn't know if my daughter and I would have a place to live. I walked into a company and was hired on the spot!

I try to get myself outdoors, by doing some hiking, taking a walk, or spending time watching animals. It makes me realize that there is an expansive world out there, and helps me gain perspective on what I am going through. Also, getting in touch with nature calms me down.

When I'm depressed or anxious, I write down both small and large blessings in a gratitude journal. This never fails to lift my spirits. Reading scripture and meditating on the promises of God is helpful. I especially like spending time in the books of *Philippians*

(*New Testament*) and *Isaiah* (*Old Testament*).

I think of my favorite quote that helped me get through a tough time. "Tough times don't last; tough people do."

Although there are many songs, here is one that is in constant rotation on my Ipod right now: "Work That" by Mary J. Blige (from her "Growing Pains" CD). This song lets you know that you will always have people who find a way to criticize, but regardless of it all, you have to realize that you are equipped with everything you need to make it through. Also, "Ain't No Stopping Sunshine" by an artist named Yoli. It was featured on the movie soundtrack "Deliver Us from Eva." This is just a feel good song that I play when I want to get pumped up. It emphasizes that regardless of external circumstances, you are in control, and should never let anyone, or anything get you down.

I do what I can. Faith really doesn't play much of a role as I look to the future more than anything else. So I suppose a healthy dose of optimism is what we need to fight it.

I've seen sunsets that have literally taken my breath away. I remember a vacation in Lake Tahoe where the sunset was so spectacular, it brought tears to my eyes, and all I could say was, "God, you did an awesome job!"

One of my favorite songs is "Calling All Angels" by Train. It seems that song is guided to my car stereo when I am having a rough time. It's as if God is sending me a message through the song, "I won't give up if you don't give up." I won't give up. God is not done with me yet.

When I think I am completely alone in this world, I look into the big, round eyes of my cat. It's hard to feel depressed when I am stroking her tummy from top to bottom as she purrs contentedly. She's my biggest fan!

I listen to my "So Sad It's Good" play list because it's good to acknowledge your feelings instead of pretending like they aren't there. I find it's helpful for me to allow myself to be sad sometimes, to be able to feel my feelings, without guilt. I know that the sooner I acknowledge it, the sooner I can say, "This too shall pass." Bad situations never last forever. I don't wallow in the sadness too long. Later, I listen to my "Feel Good Mix" and jump on my bed and force a smile. The smile eventually becomes real!

I hug my mom for a couple of minutes and really soak it in. Hugs are healing because touch and connecting with people are healing.

I lay in my hammock and allow myself to think through why I'm feeling this way or I get lost in nature. The expanse of it all, the beauty and majesty of it all, help me to put things in perspective. My issues, although they seem great to me, in the great scheme of things, many of them don't matter.

I think, "Everything works out in the end. If it hasn't worked out, it isn't the end."

I sit down and journal everything that is good in my life. I write down what I'm grateful for. This does the most to help me get out of my slump.

I ask myself, "Am I trying to please people? Am I trying to make everybody happy? What will make me happy in this situation?" And I do that thing regardless of everyone else's opinion.

I take a brisk walk. It's a no-fail way to clear my head and get back to being more positive. If it's before noon and I'm getting serotonin and vitamin D from the sun, that is even better.

I pray. I can't prove my God is real but my experience of comfort when I pray is, so I remind myself that I can't control everything and that's okay. If it's not in my control, I surrender and stop worrying about it. If it's in my control, I take action. I listen to this song: "You Never Let Go" by Matt Redman.

I cuddle with my dog. It comforts me to be around an animal who is forever loyal and loving.

I take a nap. Sometimes stress builds up because I lack sleep and my body has too many stress hormones and not enough good hormones.

I drink water and lay down, face up on my bed, close my eyes, and breathe deeply. The water is energizing and clears my head. The deep breathing helps me to slow down and refocus on the positive.

I take a dance class like hip-hop or salsa. When you're feeling sexy, it's hard to feel depressed!

I find the one person I feel like I can be completely transparent with, and I vent as openly and honestly as I can.

I hop in the shower, get dressed up in an outfit that I feel and look good in, and put on my makeup. I call up a friend and go out dancing or walk downtown.

I get a massage and focus on the way it feels instead of what I'm dealing with. I remind myself that things always run their course, with or without me.

I shift gears, stop focusing on the past (which is what depresses a lot of people) and the future (which is what makes people anxious) and live in the moment. I think this is the single most important thing to do: change your perspective. I ask myself, "What can I do right now that makes me happy?"

I get rid of expectations for good or bad and try to focus on the present experience as it unfolds. Most peoples' disappointments come because of failed expectations. If you don't expect something, you won't get disappointed. I remind myself to take situations and people as they are.

If I'm depressed about something that I had control over but messed up on, I stop my negative thought process and ask myself, "Would I say those things to a friend?" I try to be kinder to myself and treat myself the way I would treat a good friend. I remind myself that I need love, forgiveness, grace, and kindness from myself as much as my friends do.

I get out of the house and smile at cute strangers.

I take a long, brisk walk outdoors, preferably where I can get away from vast expanses of concrete and buildings. Something about breathing the fresh air, getting my blood pumping, and seeing the natural world that is so much bigger than my personal problems helps to put everything into perspective. That's my favorite short-term cure for depression.

I take a five minute "art break" to enjoy my favorite piece of art. It refreshes my eyes and my mental attitude.

Ask yourself, what are the things you've always wanted someone to say to you, but no one ever has. Then, say those things to yourself again and again. I ask the child inside of me what it needs to hear me say to it. Get comfortable saying "I Love You" to yourself and say it many times each day.

I stop and appreciate myself for every thought and act of kindness.

Make a recording (on your phone or on your computer, perhaps) or call your own voice mail/answering machine. Tell yourself the things you've always wanted your parent to say to you. Include everything you need to hear to feel loved and appreciated. Listen to the recording every day. Add to it when you think of anything else you want to hear.

I journal regularly, especially noting the self-hating ways I speak to myself. Then I make a decision to treat myself differently. Remind yourself that you were taught to treat yourself this way, and remind yourself of your commitment to treating yourself with unconditional love and acceptance, starting right now.

I walk my dog.

I buy myself a paint by number kit at the Dollar Store and spend the morning creating a little arts and crafts project. I am not an artist, by any means. Painting by numbers gives me a respite from my worry. Focusing on the details puts my mind in another place and my anxiety lessens.

I shoot photography to capture what my feelings or my depression looks like.

I think of at least one loving thing to do for myself each day.

I like to make cookies or a large tray of lasagna. I take it to one of the local firehouses. Their appreciative smiles and hugs lift my spirits right away.

I find I need to purposely make time in my busy life to sit with a cup of decaf Earl Grey in my library. I need to be quiet and listen to what my heart is trying to tell me. Though I may cry, I often feel much better, because I've been able to take the time to be with me, to think about me, to ask me what I need, to listen to me.

I read, voraciously, usually something lighthearted or funny. Pulp fiction is great for this, especially when you can suspend reality and put yourself in a character's shoes who has such ridiculous or serious problems that yours become so much less.

I take a walk around the neighborhood, to see what's new. If I'm mad or upset, I walk quickly, until I feel better, whether it's five minutes or fifty. If I'm just melancholy, I'll walk slower, trying to focus on what might have changed or the feeling of walking.

I spend time with friends, either quietly or not.

This year has been difficult. My best friend and I have been watching the complete seasons of Gilmore Girls to help lighten things up. The series made me feel loved, especially during those times that I didn't want to talk.

I go to the airport and watch families reunite at the end of the concourse. It always makes me happy that I do have my family. My children are young. Hopefully, one day, I'll be one of those mothers catching college age children, running into outstretched arms, at the end of the concourse.

I watch a children's movie, something like Finding Nemo, Ice Age or anything Charlie Brown. Perspective does such great things for people, and especially for me, because I find that my depression usually comes from how I view events and my choices related to those events.

I make a list of everything that's bothering me. I often get depressed when I feel overwhelmed by having too many things to do. Getting them on paper literally takes the clutter out of my mind and puts it on paper, where I can see it and organize it. Then I can relax and, when I feel up to it, begin to tackle one thing at a time.

I am a certified and experienced grant proposal writer. I sit and reflect on what kind of cause, charity or group needs assistance the most. I then work on the goal of making that impact happen.

I crochet an afghan, scarf, hat, tablecloth, or bedspread. This is very soothing for my soul. When I feel anxious or depressed, knitting is not so relaxing, because it is too noisy and nerve-racking if you drop a stitch.

I love mountains and whenever I feel depressed or anxious, I make a mental image of a beautiful mountain scene and imagine that I am there. It is so soothing. Also, I try to paint a landscape scene with watercolors.

I smile, even when I don't feel like it! A simple behavior such as a smile can go a long way towards convincing oneself that everything is fine. Studies have found that our conscious minds can only think of one thing at a time. If we focus on a positive behavior such as smiling, and if we associate this smile with a positive thought, such as "I am okay," we will dispel the negative thoughts from our minds and, consequently, the negative biofeedback from our bodies.

I use the practice of conscious breath (a breath practice of deep aware breathing) to help me feel my connection to everything and everyone around me. It alleviates both the psychological experiences of feeling depressed or anxious as well as the physical causes. It is so effective I merely need three breaths in this manner to come back to my expression of happiness.

I have more spirit now that I am in recovery.

I take a *Chicken Soup for the Soul* book from my personal book-shelf and go to a nursing home. I ask if there is anyone who would like to have someone read them a story. It takes me out of my self-pity. I always leave feeling much better than when I entered the nursing home.

I play a game of Scrabble with myself or a friend.

When bad things happen, I tell myself that I have the strength, and courage to get through this.

I pray for resolve to stand by my decisions, even when others think I am doing the wrong thing.

"I eat a pint of Ben and Jerry's "Cherry Garcia" every night as I watch Dr. Phil! Or, I take a hot bath while simultaneously eating a bowl of "Chunky Monkey." Or, I start each morning with a strong cup of tea and Tastykakes 'white with the chocolate stripe'. Sense a theme here?

How I Build Myself Up When I Am Not Feeling Good Enough

We all have days when we feel we are just not measuring up. Of course, we are all good enough, just the way we are! We posted a message on the Internet asking people to send in ideas. We want you to know that you are not alone. Others understand that feeling, too. So in their own unique ways, here are some of the things that other folks do when they are not feeling good enough.

WHEN I AM NOT FEELING GOOD ENOUGH

I like to read this quote from Nelson Mandela, "Our deepest fear is not that we are inadequate. Our deepest fear is that we are powerful beyond measure. It is our light, not our darkness that most frightens us. We ask ourselves, who am I to be brilliant, gorgeous, talented, fabulous? Actually, who are you not to be? Your playing small does not serve the world. There is nothing enlightened about shrinking so that other people won't feel insecure around you. We are all meant to shine, as children do. We were born to make manifest the glory of God that is within us. It's not just in some of us; it's in everyone. And as we let our own light shine, we unconsciously give other people permission to do the same. As we are liberated from our own fear, our presence automatically liberates others."

When I am feeling not good enough, I build myself up again by telling myself that that everyone feels this way at one time or another, tomorrow is a new day and I'm smart, I'm unique, and I can do anything.

I tell myself that I don't need to be perfect, I just need to be me.

The moment you let someone know how much they make a dif-ference...they do. So I tell myself, "Hey, Mark, you really make a difference!"

I ponder the quote, which I keep on my desk: "Nothing happens but first a dream."

When we finally realize that we are the I AM in the I AM, we are all connected. You can't mess up love. I remind myself to love myself.

I tell myself that being an individual is like being a pearl. I am a pearl, and I can be a truly shining light in lifting the human spirit of others (by doing good works).

When my negative, critical voice takes over my brain, I tell myself that I am special and unique. And there is no one out there in the world like me. I need to surround myself with people who encourage me to be me.

I build myself up by saying, "Look out for others." Literally, look OUT and see how you can help or be helped by others. It takes the focus off of your body and allows you to focus on the soul. Here is where all the answers lie. Ironically, you must look out to look within.

My husband loves me just the way I am.

I "hit on myself," not physically, but in a sense, flirt with myself in the mirror. I don't know when I started doing it, but I perfected it while working as a social worker in a home for sexually abused teenage girls. Many of them had horrible selfesteem problems and I would make them give themselves one compliment in the mirror before they left the house.

Self-esteem is essential in facing each new day with a spirit of creativity and adventure. Self-defeating thoughts need to be re-leased and replaced with positive self-affirmations. I like statements such as, "I now attract the resources I need. I now honor and respect who I am. I now release the past to face my future with hope."

Self-affirmations coupled with touching a relevant part of the body (like the upper mid-chest that connects to the thymus, of the immune system) create a needed mind-body integration to anchor affirmations such as, "I am lovable and capable," or "I am very important."

Rather than attempting to build myself up, I learned to allow myself to directly experience the thoughts and beliefs that were present.

When I start feeling that not good enough loop and recognize it, I tell myself, "Wait, that's a lie. It's simply not true. I'm more than good enough for my wife and family. God loves me and He is greater than my heart."

I tell myself, "It is my job here on earth to make the most of my existence. The universe loves me, and I love myself." People should never beat themselves up—the world will try to do that. We should be our own best friends.

When I feel not good enough, the problem is coming from chatter in my head. And I choose not to go to battle with "negative" chatter. Instead I take a deep breath. I connect to my body. I feel the life that is pulsing inside me. When I do that, I feel the magnificence of being alive. Feeling the pleasure of my body does more for me than any thoughts in my head.

I tell myself that I am more than I appear to be; all the world's strength and power rest inside me.

I am more than I am demonstrating!

I remind myself of a quote by Muhammad Ali, "To be a great champion, you must believe that you are the best!"

I build myself, up again by telling myself, it doesn't matter what I think. God made me for a specific purpose, and I am on the right path.

I deserve it!

It's not about feeling; it's about doing. It is easier to act yourself into a better way of feeling than to feel yourself into a better way of acting.

I am the light of God, capable of doing anything I put my mind to. Then, I visualize myself glowing with white light.

When I was young, I had a less than supportive environment and battled with depression and self-doubt quite a bit. I turned things around by picturing in my mind the life I wanted to have. And I found little ways each day to work towards it. Accomplishing little tasks helped keep me interested, on course, and they gave me results I could measure.

Somebody once told me, "When you are going through hell, you've got to keep going."

Do one day at a time, one minute at a time, one task at a time. Lots of other people have done what I'm trying to do. There's

no reason I can't do it, too. How can I find out what they did?

I am whole, complete, and perfect, just the way I am right now. I move forward with eager anticipation. I easily see the good in every situation. I deserve happiness. I claim it right now. I am well, strong, and vital. I am buoyant, happy, and free.

DNA = I am unique! I already have everything it takes to succeed. I can lift myself up, by realizing that I am like no other person on earth, given the opportunity to shine, to rise up, to make a difference, to help others, to create possibilities, to laugh, and to be happy.

Life is short, and if I choose, I can make every second count. Never give up the chance to do better, to reach higher, or to

make someone else's life happier.

I choose to give life a chance. I choose to try harder. I choose to be what only I can be!

Snatch life up and make it mine! Quit pouting and get over yourself.

I recommend the book *Anatomy of an Illness* by Norman Cousins. It's not about depression but about a serious, painful illness that he cured with his own brand of Humor Therapy. It offers hope that there are options even after the doctors give up. Try humor therapy. Four hundred years ago the author of

Gulliver's Travels said, "The three best doctors in the world are Dr. Diet, Dr. Quiet, and Dr. Merryman."

(1 John 3:19-20) By this we shall know that we originate with the truth, and we shall assure our hearts before Him as regards whatever our hearts may condemn us in, because God is greater than our hearts and knows all things.

Remember your secret agent mission is to be all of who you are. I benefited from the book, *"Self Talk, Soul Talk: What to Say When You Talk to Yourself"* by Jennifer Rothschild and Robin

McGraw.

My girls are watching how I react. I tell them when I am feeling fragile and need to come up with a plan—then I do it.

What I teach my clients when "The Enough Factor" is the issue is to post positive affirmations in the bathroom, car, wallet, or on a desk, and anywhere they go daily...I am Good Enough, I have Enough Money, I am Pretty Enough, etc.

Just as Nathaniel Branden once taught me in his books, "...the battle was lost when you, a long time ago, decided you weren't good enough, and would spend the rest of your life trying to be, in a word, GOOD, always trying in all sorts of ways to compensate for feeling intrinsically BAD. The solution: the more you trust yourself in life and build up true self-confidence, the more it feels natural to implicitly feel good, without any reason. You can give up trying to counteract a feeling that is best nipped in the bud." (This is not a literal quote; just my summary/memory of his teachings, interwoven with my own life experience and insight.)

I am perfect as God made me.

I build myself up by reading (Romans 5:8) "But God commandeth His great love toward us, while we were yet sinners, Christ died for us." I love this scripture because it tells me that I do not have to be perfect. As a matter of fact, it was while I was already a mess, and did not even acknowledge Christ, and not even born yet, He loved me so much that he gave His life for a sinner like me so that I now have the right to be called a Child of God.

What Money Can't Buy

I posed this question on the Internet and requested people send me their thoughts in response to, "Can you send me your ideas about what money can't buy." When you are feeling down, perhaps these thoughts will give you pause about the old adage—the best things in life are free!

WHAT MONEY CAN'T BUY

- Peace of mind.

- The knowledge of a job well done.

- Satisfaction.

- Serenity.

- Inspiration.

- Time with your grandchildren.

- Soaking up the sunshine on a warm spring day.

- The sharp air on your nose on a freezing cold morning in the country.

- Inner peace.

- Happiness.

- Confidence.

- Health.

- "Eternal" youth.

- Salvation.

- Money can't buy time or bring back the past.

- The feeling I get when my infant son falls asleep in my arms in the evening.

- The smile in your heart that comes when a four year old says, "You smell like vanilla. I love you!"

- Bringing back a loved one who has died.

- Returning to that moment in time, and the wisdom to use it well.

- Perfect foresight.

- Window shopping.

- Playing dress up with your best friend or daughter.

- A beautiful day at the beach.

- A dolphin sighting (depending on where you live).

- A deer sighting. I once saw a bobcat outside my house in the Santa Monica canyons. It was the most amazing thing I've ever seen.

- Laughing hysterically with your friends.

- A kiss.

- Dancing in the rain.

- Thinking right before you spoke words that while forgiven, will never be forgotten.

- Love of a spouse or child.

- A beautiful sunset or sunrise.

- Birds chirping on a spring day.

- The feeling of lying on your back in the grass on a spring or summer day.

- A hayride in the fall.

- The joy of watching kids play baseball on a summer evening.

- A harvest moon rising on an October evening.

- The cry of your firstborn grandchild.

- A drink of cool water on a hot summer day.

- Friendship.

- Respect of your peers.

- Knowing I have four people in the world who love me unconditionally.

- The ability to change myself.

- Physical and emotional health.

- Knowing myself and all my faults.

- My sanity.

- Confidence.

- A hug.

- Vitality.

- Tenacity.

- Seeing and hearing.

- My wife, who loves me, despite all of my faults.

- Vigilance.

- Perseverance.

- An open mind.

- A youthful attitude.

- Love, hope, peace, joy, support.

THE BEST THINGS IN LIFE ARE FREE!

I come home and am greeted by eight house dogs running, barking, wiggling, and waggling.

You might be able to buy the company of friends, but you'll never be able to buy their trust.

As soon as my parrot sees me, my parrot gives me this HAPPY SCREAM. There is nothing like this and I wouldn't miss it for anything in the world.

Replacement of a lost species that we failed to appreciate before it was gone.

You can't buy being spiritually grounded. A book, retreat, or workshop might point the direction, but being grounded entails sidestepping your ego.

Integrity and personal authenticity which originate from the uniqueness of your being.

You can't buy a "re-do" for past moments of your life.

Money can't be used to bring back the father who I dearly loved after passing away from a silent heart attack during my freshman year in college. After going through this experience, it has truly taught me to live every day like it is my last. The greatest things in life aren't things. They are the things you can't see. Because in the end, when all is said and done, the only things that will move on with us after we have passed are the love and relationships between everyone we loved and cared about. Material things become meaningless.

I went into the hospital thinking I was having a heart attack. Fortunately, it was just gallstones. I was put on morphine. While it took care of the pain, it caused problems with my anti-depression medicine. I'm smart enough to understand how I am feeling, but REALLY hate anxiety and feeling of doom. My saving grace is that I work with a great group. When I returned to work after being released from the hospital, I received so many wonderful hugs. My friends and their hugs have truly helped me deal with my anxiety and depression.

Reconciliation: After a very hard divorce, with a lot of fighting and destructive behavior, my ex-husband got cancer, a very rare and difficult to cure cancer. I decided to go visit him and close our story together by asking for his forgiveness and offering mine for all the negative things we did to each other. He could not talk, and was crying and pressing my hand very hard, and smiling at the same time. After two hours, I left with a wonderful feeling that money can't buy....ever.

A beautiful summer day in the middle of January—a weekend spent hiking along the California coast and reading on the beach. No better therapy after a tough week.

The feeling of love you get when your dog crawls into the crook of your body while you're sleeping.

Young children enjoying the satisfaction of learning how to tie their shoes, or counting out the proper change.

A career that I love. I am a freelance writer/editor. I bound out of bed at 5 AM, eager to start another day of work. I work seven days a week (OK, five days and two more-than-half days) by choice. I've been saying for years, there is no one in the world I'd want to trade places with!

Those warm, rosy, sleepy cheeks a toddler has when he gets up from a nap. Heaven.

The feeling of freedom when you finally learn that you gain control when you give up control!

The exhilaration of riding your bicycle in winter in southeast Florida.

The thrill of cruising along the ocean with the sun on your face and the wind at your back. It's just another day in Paradise.

True friendship, the kind that empathizes with you when you suffer a personal setback, or cries with you when you have to put your kitty-cat down.

The deep appreciation that develops between two people who have pledged their love, and committed to share and grow a life together, lasting decades, and sustained as a loving couple.

The unconditional love of a dog.

The love of a parent for a child. (And the reverse is also true.)

Gratitude. The words "thank you" lift the spirit and create a sense of harmony in our souls!

The genuine and exuberant affection and love that children give. No matter how stressful my day can be, when my daughter wraps her arms around me with unconditional love, I know I am truly blessed and grateful.

Waking up at dawn on a backpacking trip. The first smile of the morning from a baby. The sound of a rain under a metal awning. A great morning snuggle.

Self control.

The sound of babies giggling.

The crunch of snow under my feet on a winter walk. A warm bed when my toes are cold.

The ability to rhyme and sing with ease. Holding hands all the way to school. Catching snowflakes on my tongue.

My ability to affect change in others.

Digging snow forts.

Helping someone out with no expectation of reciprocation. The first snow of the season.

The last snow of the season.

Waking up to kisses—first my sweetie, then my dogs. Warm tea.

The sun shining in my face. Crossing things off my to-do list.

Getting more done today than yesterday. Quiet!

The silence of snowfall.

Sleeping puppies, feet and mouths twitching. A letter, by mail from a friend.

New leaves on a plant that was dying. Waking up rested and refreshed.

Hot shower. Sunset.

The feeling of fulfillment or contentment. That feeling comes from within, and it touches on so many areas.

Health for your children.

Making you a nice person. Some wealthy people are actually quite selfish.

The unexpected joy from dancing to music in the privacy of your own home.

The calming effect of spending time to connect with your center through journaling.

Sharing your experiences with someone who really listens. And feeling truly heard.

The satisfaction of having taken good care of yourself by choosing to eat healthy, nourishing, and delicious food.

The feeling of ease after finally filing that mountain of papers on your desk. (Feel free to substitute "Filing papers" with cleaning the toilet, vacuuming under your bed, paying that parking ticket...)

The feeling of release after fully expressing your anger, either to the party that deserves it, or in the privacy and safety of your own home.

The empowering feeling that follows saying "no" or "yes."

That feeling of satisfaction of coming back from working out, especially if you didn't feel like going, in the first place.

The inkling of hope that arises after you make a list of what you want your life to look like, and choosing one thing to change.

The effects: physically, mentally, emotionally, of a hearty belly laugh.

The relief that comes from a job well done, or a project that is finally completed.

A few minutes of solitude—total solitude—in an otherwise hectic day.

Satisfaction in completing a jigsaw puzzle, a crossword puzzle, a Sudoku puzzle, or any puzzle.

Watching a baby or a tot learn how to walk, mesmerized by the world around them.

Good taste, dignity, compassion, attentiveness, listening skills, integrity, balance in life.

The smell of the air after it rains. The sound of children's laughter.

When clouds look like angels, or animals. When my son or husband says, "I love you." Walking around the farmers' market. Waking up breathing in the morning.

A hot shower.

Laying under a shady tree on a sunny day.

The way the fog makes everything quiet and still. Hearing an owl hoot at night.

A boyfriend who cracks the ice on your front stoop with a hammer so you won't fall—without you even asking him to do it. (Scene: The gutter on our townhouse is frozen and wa-ter is dripping down onto our front stoop creating a smooth sheet of ice. My boyfriend has just walked in and commented on it. Conversation:

My roommate (jokingly): We should crack it with a hammer.

My boyfriend (to me): Do you have a hammer?

Me: Yes, but you don't have to do that. I can do it later. My boyfriend: It will take 5 minutes. Just give me the hammer.

He goes outside, and in five minutes our treacherous stoop is clear.)

The ability to play a musical instrument. I play clarinet and sax. When people used to say to me, "I wish I could play sax," I'd say, "Get one and I'll teach you." Later, I realized that they didn't want to learn; they just wanted to be able to play without having to practice.

The sound of the person you love most saying "*I love you.*" Hearing people laugh.

A good marriage that is about love, friendship, caring, and support to muster through the rough times. We have different ways of coping with challenges. We take the best of what we do and it becomes a good mix to go forward with optimism.

Adaptability and resiliency and the ability to change with circumstances.

A Conscience. Common Sense. Talent.

The smell of the ocean where I grew up—I cannot duplicate it. The sounds of my children playing, wrestling, laughing, whining!

The memory of my first date with my husband. I knew I would marry him when he would not kiss me goodnight!

The thrill of finding a longlost friend on Facebook and discovering that you both have not aged so gracefully!

The taste of Rombauer Chardonnay—it is the best ever! Crackling wood in the fireplace.

Getting a good rest or sleeping well throughout the night! The satisfaction of owning my own business.

Knowing that when I go to bed at night, that the three people I love the most are no more than 20 feet from me.

The nook—the place where I rest my head on my husband's chest at night—no one else can buy that!

The warm satisfaction you feel after performing a random act of kindness.

Spontaneous laughter at a well-told joke.

A sense of accomplishment at the successful conclusion of a project.

Your faithful dog's greeting when you come home from work.

Realizing you've forgotten the world exists because you've been playing with your grandchild.

Thoughtfulness and the knowledge and feeling that someone is thinking of you.

Our memories of my father. My dad always had a toothpick in his mouth, when he kissed mom, when he went into surgery, when he walked me down the aisle, and when he talked with customers at the post office. Even during his death, he had his toothpick. So when dad sold me his car, and I found the toothpick he had hidden in the car (to say he was thinking of me), I tucked it in my pocket. Each time I feel that toothpick, I do something in his honor. Dad died over five years ago; I still have the toothpick he left for me; I continue to "pay it forward" in his honor.

Personal power, that comes from the inside, from allowing ourselves to stand up proudly and show the world what we are really made of. Mother Teresa didn't have money, but she had power. Many of the world's wealthy would listen to her and do as she asked. Gandhi didn't use money to change the face of India. He used his voice and his strength of conviction and that inspired people. Money just can't buy that time with your wife and children.

Playing a board game as a family on Friday evening, or going to a movie together.

Taking back a mean or rude comment to someone.

The pride I have about my two children, both young men and both in college. They have grown into kind, caring, and loving young adults. Both call me on a regular basis just to tell me "stuff." My son sent me an e-mail saying he is proud to be my son. My youngest texts and calls me often about issues he's dealing with at school and asking my opinion. Every night I say my own version of a prayer, thanking whomever it is that gave me these two wonderful people. I know that I am "paying it forward" because they are growing into caring adults with warm hearts. In fact, my oldest told me once he can't wait to be a father because it must be so much fun to have kids. Although their dad divorced me, the two good things that came out of the marriage are these two boys. Money could never buy me the happiness that my boys bring me.

When I became a grandma eight years ago. I never imagined the joy I would find in one tiny little being. Money can't buy that joy. And neither can money buy a grandchild's sweet kiss, nor a hug that doesn't even go all the way around. Money can't buy a grandchild's innocent question. Or eyes that dance when you walk into a room. I've been blessed with eight more grandchildren. Yes, nine of them. I am the wealthiest woman in the entire world, and I haven't spent a dime for it!

Your thoughts, faith, your will, creativity, the sky, the ocean, the stars, grace, and stillness.

Hearing your favorite song on the radio. A hug when you really need one.

Finding something you thought you'd lost a long time ago. My kid saying something hilarious and laughing until I cry. A sunny day when you have plans to go outdoors.

My husband making a difference. My husband was an officer with an upward, yet unfulfilling career. While spending a year in the Middle East, he watched lives changed forever by the war, families changed forever by the loss of their soldiers, and saw the need to invest in one's own family while there is still opportunity. Even though he liked the military and supported the global war on terror, he put in his paperwork to get out of active duty, and he became involved on a day-to-day basis at the school where our children attend. Every day he is there with them, investing in their lives and education! His salary is maybe one-fourth of what he made before, but the satisfaction of making a difference is worth so much more than money!

Sitting in a comfortable chair in a sunny window on a cold winter's day reading a favorite book, while drinking a cup of hot tea, with my dog in my lap.

Being married to a wonderful spouse. Having a job that you love going to. Your little girl saying "I love you, Daddy." Watching the leaves change color in the fall. Inspiring others to handle their finances better. Making a difference in the world by teaching students.

The look on my new granddaughter's face when she is smiling up at me. The song in my heart as I watch my children with their children. The peace in the room when my husband and I are communicating without even speaking.

Understanding, sense of humor, memories, confidence, your soul, spirituality.

The conversation between best girlfriends that bring tears of laughter.

The look on a child's face when they first learn how to read.

A Game Night, either with friends or a multigenerational family. You can't buy the energy and spirit that happens when groups play and laugh together. A deck of cards can get the party started and maybe some Cheetos (or organic blue corn chips and brie, depending on the crowd).

Inner peace-centering during Yoga or meditation is something you can't buy in any store.

The love of a child is something that cannot be bought, only earned.

Having a passion for what you do, whether it's business or just for fun.

Enjoying beautiful scenery, taking a walk in nature, a sunset, a garden, or the view from the top of a mountain.

Learning about who you are from the inside out and celebrating what makes you unique.

Your interests, talents, gifts, way of looking at things and expressing them are all priceless.

A sense of humor. I've been married to my sweet husband for more than eight years and he still makes me laugh so hard my stomach hurts. Whether he is talking to people on TV (as if they can hear him), quoting movie lines or just plain being goofy, his sense of humor makes me fall in love with him every time I laugh.

A life free of uncertainty—nor should we want it to! Uncertainty causes a lot of anxiety, but it's also part of the joy of being alive.

Imagination.

Trust—that's hard-earned and easily lost. Forgiveness (or forgetfulness, for that matter).

A baby's smile or a child's hug. Looking up on a clear night and seeing an infinite star field. Sitting in a public library, reading all the latest magazines Taking a ride on the swings at your local playground.

A kiss on the cheek from your kid as she leaves for school.

A new paradigm, a new way of thinking. With all of the problems in the world, we are finding that money cannot buy our way out. In order to change our world, we have to change our way of thinking and money just does not do that. Perhaps it is the lack of money that will help turn the tide.

My faith—the one thing I truly own that can not be bought or stolen, it does not rust, and no one has enough money that could ever replace what it provides me.

Watching the sun rise—anywhere.

Blowing on a dandelion and watching the wind carry the spores away like little parachutes.

Listening to a chorus of third graders singing Christmas carols. The smell of chocolate chip cookies coming from the oven.

The feeling you get from doing something nice for a stranger without being asked.

The great clean feeling after a warm shower on a cold day. The giggle of a small child.

The cooing of a baby when they smile at you. A cuddle from someone you love.

A smile from a stranger when you help them in some way (get up to give them your seat, open the door for them, carry their groceries across a street, help them with a jacket).

A garden of sunflowers smiling at you in the sun. Walking in the rain.

Sledding down a hill in your local neighborhood. Popping in to a friend's house for a coffee and chat. A note from a friend reminding you they care.

A poem from history that is as relevant today as it was when it was written.

Cheering for a child at sports and watching their face light up when they know you are there.

Laughing at yourself singing in the shower. Laughing so hard your sides hurt.

The feeling of listening to the song 'Ave Maria', 'Amazing Grace', and 'How Great Thou Art.'

The feeling of being productive. It has always been my pet peeve to be a warm body in a chair, no matter how much an employer was paying me, because they could never repay my time wasted in "presenteeism". That is one bright side to this economic downturn—now everyone left standing will be expected to pitch in and do more than they were hired to do.

Erasing the mistakes. Money can only buy tangibles. But satisfaction in one's accomplishments, making mistakes, and life........

They come through the journey we all make, and must make until our end whatever that may be.

A walk in the woods, when snow is tumbling down and muting the outside noise, so all you hear are your footsteps.

Love. It feels nice and warm on a cold winter morning.

Support from your peers and the drive to give back. I believe that knowing there is going to be a better tomorrow can be a motivation to "stay in the fight" and being part of that type of community, knowing you've made a difference, can be the path to recovery.

What to Do When You Are Sad, Blue, Anxious, Down in the Dumps and You Don't Even Want to Get Up in the Morning

We placed this posting on the Internet. When people are feeling down, hopeless, stressed, or depressed, they need some "pick-me-uppers." Any suggestions for happy movies to watch, one line quotes that inspire hope, books to read, songs, things to do that will lift their spirits? The ideas below are sure to spark creative ways to chase the blues away. Here are some "quick pick-me-ups," expressed just as folks shared them with us.

PICK-ME-UPS

When my problems seem like the weight of the world is on my shoulders, I go outside to look at a breathtaking sunset or watch the moon as it plays Hide and Seek among the clouds. Seeing the vastness of this Universe makes my problems seem so small in comparison.

I suggest that you keep a **Journal of Acknowledgments**, to really acknowledge yourself for all the good and positive things you *have* done vs. those you beat yourself up for not doing. An example of an Acknowledgment statement would be: *I acknowledge myself for not eating all that was on my plate at dinner, and stopping when I felt satisfied* (great for people with emotional eating/dieting issues.*)*

I take a walk and "breathe in" the colors around me: the trees, plants, flowers, houses, cars. This keeps me present and grounded. It fills me up with appreciation of my world.

I do a brain dump! This means sitting with pen and paper and writing whatever thoughts or feelings are going through you without judgment or criticism. Just write for 3 pages or 20 minutes; whichever comes first. There is generally a sense of release and relief at the end so that you can move forward.

I watch or listen to a favorite comedian for 30 minutes (longer if you have the time) and just laugh out loud.

I turn some of my favorite music on and just dance for 45 seconds. I tell people who "can't" dance, just to move their arms and feet and jump around. This will change anyone's mood in a matter of seconds, make you smile and make you forget what you were down about in the first place.

Watch the movies "The Pursuit of Happyness" or "Facing the Giants."

There is a beautiful song by Jon & Vangelis called "I'll Find My Way Home"—very uplifting!

I keep a "First Aid Kit" handy. It's a cheapie little metal lunch box I bought at the dollar store years ago. Inside I have a photo of my best friend and me with big cheesy grins on our faces. This photo reminds me I have people to call when I'm down.

When I am down for a while I start chanting to myself: "I am glad that I am so great and everything always turns out for me!" And you know what? If I say that with enough feeling and enough times, I start getting better right away

In response to your request for a "pick-me-upper", I have a bird feeder at my window, the kind with suction cups so it's literally on my window. I can't help but smile when the sparrows jockey for space on the feeder.

I write a letter of appreciation to someone. Forget yourself and do something for someone else. Feeling disconnected, alone, or powerless makes us blue. Giving to others makes us feel more con-nected, less alone, more self-confident, and more in control. And the gift doesn't have to cost anything. Research at the University of Pennsylvania found that writing (and delivering) a letter of appreciation to someone boosted happiness higher than anything else, including splurging on oneself or indulging in a special treat.

Watch Comedy Central or You Tube. Google funny animals videos and see what shows up. You will be howling with laughter.

I'm a big advocate of writing every day in a gratitude journal. Mine is a simple Word document, and I just go to the end, put in today's date and try to list 5-10 things I'm thankful for. I often list very simple things, "I'm thankful that the sun is shining," "I'm thankful my house has heat," "I'm thankful for my children," "I'm thankful for running water." It can be that simple because you immediately become aware of how many people have no house, no heat, no children, no water, etc. and you start feeling very fortunate and that life is quite good.

Listen to: "Encourage Yourself" by Donald Lawrence, "Can't Give Up Now" by Mary, Mary and "Impossible Dream" sung by Luther Vandross.

Watch DVDs: "The Secret", "What the Bleep?", "Celestine Prophesy"

Watch Movies: "Lord of the Rings", "Star Wars", "Chronicles of Narnia", Harry Potter series.

Watch Music DVD: Sarah Brightman Read Poetry: Hafiz "The Gift"

Jack Canfield: "Chicken Soup for the Soul" books

Read "Excuse Me Your Life is Waiting." I just saw your request for pick me ups. I love the song "Always Look on the Bright Side of Life," from Monty Python's "Life of Brian" and "Spamalot". It always makes me smile!

Going for a walk helps. If I go out for at least 15 minutes, I come back feeling better.

Watch Comedy Central on television and laugh. Visit Deepak Chopra's web site. I find when I do this the first thing in the morning, the day goes much better.

Something I started when I was in my 20's... when I would get a written compliment or thank you from someone, I would put it in a file. Or if someone told me how I had made a difference in their life, I would put it on a note and put it in the file. Then when I would get down, I could pull out the file and remember why I do what I do and remember my value. I would also put motivational sayings or things that touched my heart. Articles of inspiration or quotes... It would help me get through times when I didn't feel I could go on or felt like what I was doing didn't make a difference. As a manager, with each new employee I would start a file for them and make sure I had something for them to put in it and teach them to build their own files.

I have a box that contains a lot of my favorite things: In it, I have a photo of a friend and me when we were young kids—we're leaning back on branches in an apple tree. That photo reminds me of youth and carefree feelings. It reminds me I used to climb trees. I have a picture from my wedding which is a favorite photo of my hubby and me. It reminds me that I am so loved. I have lots of pictures of my two kids. It reminds me that I have people to love. I also have some chocolate (in case of emergency). So I look at old photos and eat chocolate!

I have a disc of upbeat songs that tend to always cheer me up. I have some Wild Strawberry Bubble Gum (insanely sugary but it tastes like childhood and it's hard to feel depressed when you're blowing a bubble the size of your head).

I always keep makeup handy such as lip gloss and mascara in my purse. In case, after a hard cry, I have to look perked up.

Keep goofy items such as a Slinky and a paddle ball in the house. It is hard to feel cranky when you're focusing your energy on trying to whack that ball tied by a rubber band to a paddle.

I have a journal that I write down my blessings. Over the years I've kept a first aid kit near my nightstand. It contains lots of things that make me feel good. I grab it as needed. I don't need it often but when I do, it's nice that it is all put together—waiting for me to grab from my closet shelf. The journal is kind of neat to reread every now and then. I keep things in there that I know will make me smile.

When you are feeling down, find photos of things that make you happy and either glue them into a book or create a power point presentation that you can click through to instantly lighten your spirits. Pictures may be from someone's personal photos or even include internet pictures of cute pets, babies, beautiful land-scapes, etc. I have found that even the process of spending time finding pictures of things that you like, positively impacts mood.

How Family Members Can Fill Their Love Tank When a Loved One Is Depressed or Anxious

I want to thank all of the people on the Internet who responded to our request for tips for this section. They are all part of the team who help to encourage those coping with challenging situations. Sometimes we are "overworked" and try to do too much. Some tips came from professionals in the field and others from those "down in the trenches." When we spend so much time caring for others, we lose sight of the importance of caring for ourselves.

Talk with a friend: In person or on the phone. Talk about yourself and your needs rather than your loved one's needs.

Play games (video, computer, board games) Go outside to run, walk, bike, ride, etc. .

Talk with a counselor, privately, or in a group to get the support and compassion for what you're going through.

Take breaks! It's OK to take time away and NOT discuss the family member you're caring for! Go out for dinner, movies, coffee, a walk in the park, window shop, etc. It matters less where you go and what you do, and more that it is respite without responsibility for the moment.

Participate in physical activity: Physical activity helps recharge your emotional and physical batteries. If there is no sport you like or can participate in, how about a water aerobics class, or just a brisk walk outside, or even on a tread mill with your favorite TV show.

Rent and watch favorite movies. This can be done alone, or with friends.

Invite friends over for an evening of potluck dinner: This doesn't have to be planned long in advance, and, in fact, can be quite spontaneous to get you over a particularly rough day.

All we need to do is reach out to one another for a little support in times of need. At the end of the day we are all on the same team in this game of life and those of us that foster that idea will survive through any challenge life throws our way.

I have found that there is no greater love relationship that one can have than with oneself. When I start getting a little low on fuel, I go for a walk or hike in nature and appreciate that we are all connected and that I am a magnificent part of this world. When you do something that makes you healthier, you cannot help but feel the love.

Remember that when one person over functions, the other under functions.

Know your limits and know when you have had enough!

Reading Group Guide

No More Secrets

A Family Speaks About Depression,

Anxiety, and Attempted Suicide

Discussion Questions

What was unique about the format of the book and how did it enhance or take away from the story?

Would you consider this a fiercely candid and eyeopening account of family life when one person is diagnosed with an illness?

What would you have done if this had happened to a member of your family? Tell all or keep the secret?

What specific theme did each member of the family emphasize throughout the book? What do you think he or she is trying to get across to the reader?

Do you think school children should learn about mental health issues along with the dangers of drugs and alcohol education?

Does the family seem real and believable? Can you relate to their feelings of shame, embarrassment and secrecy? To what extent do they remind you of yourself or someone you know?

How does the family change or evolve throughout the experience? What events trigger such changes?

In what ways do the events in the book reflect what you have observed on television, radio, or print media reporting of a mental illness?

What recent current events beg the need for improved mental health programs?

Did certain parts of the book make you uncomfortable? If so, why did you feel that way? Did this lead to a new understanding or awareness of some aspect of your life you might not have thought about before?

What did you find surprising in this book?

How has reading this book changed your opinion of families dealing with mental health issues?

Do the authors present information in a way that is interesting and insightful, and if so, how do they achieve this?

Has the book increased your interest in the subject matter?

Why do you think that many families keep quiet about mental health issues?

If you were working on a campaign to end discrimination about mental health, what are three things you would do?

What are three things we can do to improve the quality of life for those affected by mental illness and their families?

We welcome your comments about the book and your thoughts pertaining to the discussion questions.

WWW.TEAMOFANGELS.COM

WWW.SPEAKINGABOUTDEPRESSION.COM

If you would like to share your thoughts, please contact: John and Patricia Gallagher

Box 561, Worcester, PA 19490

To schedule an interview or obtain a quote from the Gallaghers, please contact John at 267-939-0365 or via email *info@speakingaboutdepression.com*

A TEAM OF ANGELS
TO THE RESCUE

Patricia Gallagher of Pennsylvania, had never thought about writing devotional poems or making angel pins when she decided to launch THE SEND A TEAM OF ANGELS TO HELP MOVEMENT in 1998. She had lots of friends who were going through heartbreaking circumstances and she was facing her own special challenges. She wanted to reach out to them, as well as find a way to cope. "I started writing poems and making little team of angel pins from craft materials," she recalls. Soon, Patricia was making pins by the thousands. The campaign has distributed some 7500 pins to United States troops in the Middle East as well as wounded soldiers in military hospitals. Over 100,000 team of an-gel pins have offered comfort to people with cancer, depression, addictions, and a host of other challenges. People who receive the pins treasure them because it means someone cares. The Team of Angels alone won't solve all of the problems of the world, but the comfort they provide means a lot, and so does simply knowing that somebody is thinking of you. You can see the team of angel pins—and order a team of angels— for just ten dollars at www.teamofangels.com

To find out more about how to join the SEND A TEAM OF ANGELS TO HELP MOVEMENT or to start a TEAM OF ANGELS CHAPTER, please contact: Team of Angels, Box 561, Worcester, PA 19490

Real Dads. Real Men. Real Families. Real Depression Campaign

What do the Gallaghers share during their presentations?

John and Patricia Gallagher begin their presentation by showing a five minute news clip of the personal stories of "real men" who have suffered with depression, including a firefighter, a retired Air Force Sergeant, a lawyer, a national diving champion, a college student and a writer. They express their thanks to all who are reaching out to help as sponsors and in so doing have provided hope to others. John and Patricia communicate key messages— symptoms, recovery, where to get help—but also use active listening skills to connect with the personal experience of participants. John shares his personal story of overcoming depression. His amazing story is of recovery through faith, family support, and hope.

Is the program only suitable for men?

The program gives all people, not just men, information on how to recognize depression in friends and family members and offers men and the people who care about them a way to take the next step of seeking help.

What are the goals?

The four goals for the campaign are as follows: to reduce stigma and thereby help to prevent suicide; to promote the 1-800-SUI-CIDE Hopeline, to raise awareness that depression is a major public health problem in men and encourage families to seek help.

How did this program begin?

The campaign began when Morris J. Cohen and Company, a CPA firm and the Clayman Family Foundation offered a development grant for the purpose of bringing the campaign to organizations. Programs were enthusiastically received by the United Way Kick-Off campaign at Exelon/Limerick Power Plant, Women in Recovery, Meadow Wood Psychiatric Hospital, the New Choices Program at Montgomery County Community College, as well as many Rotary groups, schools, civic groups, and churches.

Are messages tailored for addressing depression in the workforce ?

John and Patricia Gallagher are founding partners in the *Speaking About Depression Initiative*, which aims to de-stigmatize depression and train people on the many, varied topics of depression in the workplace. Their program topic for the workplace is titled **Speaking about Depression is a Good Business Move.**

Are there programs specifically for the faith-based communities?

A special program titled *Hanging on to Faith When Life Falls Apart* is an uplifting presentation for churches, schools, retreats, spiritual and religious organizations.

Why have you also addressed the specific issues of the Asian, Latino, Gay and African-American communities?

Recognizing that diverse cultures exist in the USA, the Gallaghers partner with representatives of many backgrounds. Most cultures hold fast to beliefs that they have been taught. Many men think that it is weak or feminine if you admit to needing help. In the Asian community, there is often a "code of silence" so as not to bring shame on the family, regarding depression. In the Latino community, mental health problems and men are not considered "macho". Programs are tailored to meet diverse needs.

******

Real Dads. Real Men. Real Families. Real Depression Campaign

In addition to foundations, sponsors and corporate donors, who else would the Gallaghers like to meet?

Important to the success of the program is the active participation of key stakeholders in the community, including businessmen and women who might be willing to tell their personal stories or underwrite the cost of programs. The Gallaghers would like to meet families who might be interested in creating a foundation in memory of a loved one who committed suicide or experienced a mental illness. They would like to enlist such support for the campaign, as well as their other outreach programs.

Are volunteers needed?

Contacts and volunteers are needed to distribute posters and brochures to firehouses, police stations, sheriff's departments, jails, detention centers, community mental health organizations and recovery programs. Volunteers are needed for placing Public Service Announcements on media venues. Volunteers can raise funds, coordinate special events, provide administrative services, assist with public relations, offer legal assistance, maintain web sites, and general volunteer opportunities. **Donations of time, talent and funds are greatly appreciated.**

The Gallaghers welcome interviews and speaking engagements.

www.speakingaboutdepression.com

www.teamofangels.com

Info@speakingaboutdepression.com

John And Patricia Gallagher Are Coming To A City Near You!

They are embarking on a tour of America to speak about the message of this book, including bringing attention to the collateral damage that happens to a family when secrets are kept about depression, anxiety and attempted suicide.

Call 267-939-0365 to schedule a visit for a church, gathering, coffeehouse, library, school, support group, conference, retreat, corporation, etc.

Visit *www.speakingaboutdepression.com*

ALSO BY PATRICIA C. GALLAGHER

- ✓ *Start Your Own At-Home Child Care Business*

- ✓ *Raising Happy Kids on a Reasonable Budget*

- ✓ *So You Want to Open a Profitable Day Care Center*

- ✓ *No More Secrets – A Family Speaks about Anxiety, Depression and Attempted Suicide*

- ✓ *The Gift of a Team of Angels*

- ✓ *For All the Write Reasons – 40 Successful*

- ✓ *Authors Tell You How to Get a Book Published*

- ✓ *The Courageous and Self-Respecting Gift of Saying Goodbye - Daily Reflections for Anyone*

- ✓ *Considering Parting Ways in a Relationship and Who Needs the Strength to Let Go*

- ✓ *The Gift of Believing in Yourself –Wisdom, Observations, Suggestions, and Reminders*

- ✓ *The Pass It On Angel Pin Lady - One*

- ✓ *Suburban Mom's Effort to Pin the World Together with Angel Pins*

- ✓ *What Can God Do with a Woman Like Me?*

- ✓ *The Complete Kids' Guide to Being a Super Babysitter*

- ✓ *Christmas on Lindbergh Mountain Audio Book*

- ✓ *Granny Trisha's Play and Learn Book*

- ✓ *The Gift of Changing Yourself – Daily Thoughts for Women in Transition*

Patricia Gallagher holds a BA in Education and a MBA in Finance and Management. When Patricia Gallagher's children were young, before depression touched their family, she appeared as a guest on many shows including Oprah Winfrey, The 700 Club, CNN, CNBC, Sally Jessy Raphael, Maury Povich, Financial News Network, EWTN, and others. These appearances were related to her book *Raising Happy Kids on a Reasonable Budget,* and *Start Your Own At-Home Child Care Business*. The CBS Early Show did a segment at the Gallagher home related to the *Team of Angels* pins. She hosted a tri-state radio show, *Come Share Your Faith*.

Mail Order Form:

Step 1 — Please print out this page.

Step 2 — Fill in shipping address:

Name _____

Address _____

City _____ State _____

Zip _____ Phone_____

Email _____

Step 3 — Enter the quantity you'd like to order next to its description:

____ The Gallagher's book "**NO MORE SECRETS** - A Family Speaks About Depression, Anxiety and Attempted Suicide" $19.95 plus $7.50 shipping and handling (See book info at *www.speakingaboutdepression.com*)

____ Two team of angel lapel pins, packaged with 12 assorted poem verse book-marks $19.95 plus $7.95 shipping and handling.

____ Team of Angel lapel pins, **without the bookmarks**, $10 each plus $4.95 shipping and handling. (Just the pins!)

____ Team of Angels bookmarks, **without the team of angels pins**, are packed in quantities, of 50 assorted bookmarks $25 plus $4.95 shipping and handling.

Titles of the poems: see verses at *www.teamofangels.com* (online catalog)

____ FOR HOPE

____ OVERWHELMED

____ PROTECT MY LOVED ONES

___ FRIENDSHIP

___ THINKING OF YOU

___ SOMEONE SPECIAL

___ TO THANK YOU

___ TO PROTECT ALL MILITARY FAMILIES

___ TO THANK OUR UNITED STATES ARMED FORCES

___ GET WELL

___ SERIOUS ILLNESS

___ PEACE ON EARTH

___ DIETERS

Step 4 (PA Residents Only) — Apply 6% Sales tax to Sub-Total:

PA Sales Tax = $_____

Step 5 — Grand Total: Sub-Total + PA Sales Tax = $_____

Step 6 — Mail this form and check or money order for grand total payable to:

Patricia C. Gallagher
PO Box 561
Worcester, PA 19490

Questions and information, please call #267-939-0365

Email: *theangelpinlady@gmail.com*

Coaching Services

ABOUT THE AUTHOR

After leaving her corporate position at AT&T to care for her children at home, Patricia Gallagher decided to combine her business savvy with her love for children. She began a child care center out of her home and has turned the years of experience into fourteen books, numerous journal articles, pamphlets and publications.

Patricia holds a BA in Elementary Education and an MBA in Finance and Management and has enjoyed many professions, including elementary school teacher, college instructor, preschool director and day care mother.

Patricia has been a featured guest on the "Oprah Winfrey Show," "Sally Jessy Raphael," "Maury Povich," "People Are Talking," "Hour Magazine," Financial News Network, CNN, CNBC, The 700 Club, EWTN, The CBS Early Show, Lifetime, Interview with Joan Lunden, and many other shows. Articles about Patricia Gallagher's expertise have also been featured in over 200 national and local magazines and newspapers including the Stars and Stripes military newspaper, The Wall Street Journal and media wire services such as Gannett, UPI, Associated Press and Scripps Howard.

Patricia Gallagher lives in Pennsylvania. She is the mother of four adult children and the grandmother of one. She welcomes interviews, speaking engagements, and consultations.

Patricia C. Gallagher

www.patriciausa.com
Office: (267) 939-0365

www.ingramcontent.com/pod-product-compliance
Lightning Source LLC
Chambersburg PA
CBHW021427170526
45164CB00001B/125